SHORT-TERM
KETO

A 4-Week Plan to Find Your Unique Carb Threshold

TARA GARRISON

VICTORY BELT PUBLISHING

LAS VEGAS

Cover design by Kat Lannom

Front cover photo by Lyman Winn

Interior design by Charisse Reyes and Crizalie Olimpo

Illustrations by Eli San Juan and Allan Santos

Printed in Canada
TC 0121

CONTENTS

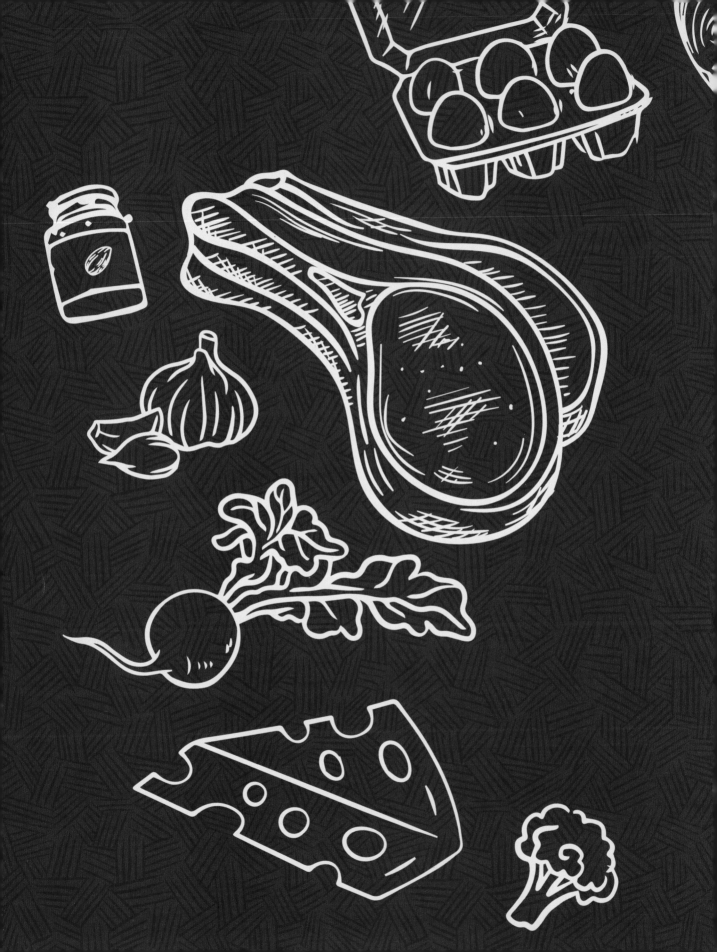

INTRODUCTION

*"It's not a short-term diet,
it's a long-term lifestyle."*

—Anonymous

I'm so excited to bring you this book that has been born out of the trenches of coaching people one-on-one through the ketogenic diet as my full-time job for the past five years.

Back in 2017, when keto was really building momentum, the message from the keto community was loud and clear: keto is the superior way for humans to eat.

While I saw the life-changing benefits of the ketogenic diet for many people, I also observed a lot of dogmatic attitudes and cultlike vibes that didn't sit well with me. I started seeing people getting their identities wrapped up in it. Labeling someone as a "fat burner" or "sugar burner" became commonplace, with the clear connotation that fat burners were superior, more educated people. Sugar burners, the people who ate carbs and ran on glucose, were somehow regarded as inferior for not understanding that "optimized" humans run on ketones. I started seeing fearmongering messages saying that carbs will inflame you—or even kill you—which created a fear of all carbohydrates, except for the "approved" keto diet–friendly vegetables.

Fear around food soon grew to an astronomical level in the keto community. All of a sudden, a huge number of people were claiming to be "carb addicts." This label made me raise an eyebrow. Addicted to a macronutrient? The macronutrient that is the primary fuel source for the human body? I didn't like what I was seeing on the mental and emotional side of things in the keto world. Labeling foods as "bad" or "prohibited" is never a healthy practice.

I was discouraged to see that even though I tried to help my clients and followers understand that carbs weren't "bad" and were to be restricted only temporarily to enhance the metabolism, people almost always developed a negative relationship with carbs anyway. For many, a vine-ripe grape and a cookie fell into the same category: bad. And because people are human and carbohydrates are delicious, when they ate one carb-rich food, they would often go completely off the rails because they "already blew it" and binge on all the foods they'd been missing. These kinds of behaviors can have a massive negative effect on a person's self-esteem and create disordered eating patterns.

All this made me ask myself, What is going on here?

I'm all for sharing information with people and giving them options for nutritional strategies that might work for them, but the messages from the keto world were not that. There was no room for questioning whether a carbohydrate-based diet might be beneficial for a person. Even hinting at it would be embarrassing. You should know better. Intelligent people know better.

The keto community became an elitist group. Keto didn't work for you? It couldn't have been keto's fault; you must not have done it right. I have seen people be bullied and kicked out of ketogenic online communities for even questioning keto. These trends seriously concerned me because, as a nutrition coach, I know the detrimental effects that this kind of thinking can have on people when they become so identified with a nutritional approach that they won't change, even if it's hurting their health.

Now let me give you some context by sharing my own keto journey.

My experience with the ketogenic diet was pretty unique in the fact that when I started, I had 11 percent body fat and was in incredible shape. Most people start keto as a weight-loss tactic or to heal something in their bodies. I didn't have either of those issues, so I was coming at it from a healthy metabolic standpoint.

When I first tried keto, I got a DEXA scan to measure my body composition. The results: 11.3 percent body fat, 122 pounds of lean mass, and 15 pounds of fat on my body. That's very lean for a woman. I had no idea I was that lean. I had just run a marathon in 3 hours 17 minutes (a per-mile pace of 7:31 minutes), qualified for the Boston Marathon, and was training heavily in the gym. I was in great shape. To get there, I had followed a higher-protein diet with low to moderate carbohydrates and low to moderate dietary fat. (Fat and carbs fluctuated; I just prioritized whole foods from nature.)

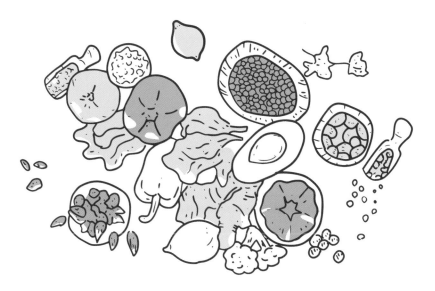

BEFORE KETO

When I was introduced to keto, I was hesitant at first. I felt like I had already found my groove in nutrition. I was a lean, mean, muscly machine—and I had accomplished that without tracking my food. But I was intrigued by and interested in the reported health benefits of keto, especially for the brain, so I decided to give it a go.

The first thing I noticed was that my mind felt better. I felt less stressed and calmer. I felt like I could think more clearly—like my whole brain had woken up. Mentally, I felt like a superhuman.

However, I also noticed that I was gaining weight. Now, I intentionally wanted to get my body fat a little higher after finding out I was at 11 percent. Ten to 12 percent is essential fat for a woman. So I purposefully indulged in more calories.

When I went back for another DEXA scan four months later, I had gained 11 pounds, about 10 of which were fat, which put me at 17 percent body fat. I was okay with that, but I definitely didn't want to keep gaining body fat at that rate; that is a lot of gain in four months! I decided I felt best at around 14 to 15 percent body fat and wanted to get back down to that range and maintain it. So I played with keto in all sorts of ways, but no matter how hard I tried, that bit of fat loss just wasn't happening. At my next scan a few weeks later, I had lost a couple of pounds, but they were from muscle mass. Four months later, after optimizing protein and post-workout nutrition, supplementing with leucine, and eating high-quality food, I scanned again only to find that I was up to 18 percent body fat and had lost 5.5 pounds of muscle mass.

So, in total, after nine months of strict keto, I had gained 10.5 pounds of fat and lost 5.5 pounds of muscle.

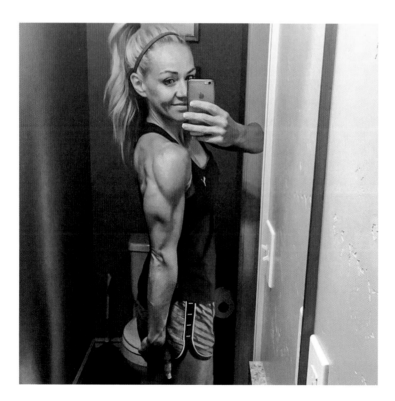

DURING KETO

What's interesting is that I chose to continue eating keto even after watching these numbers trend unfavorably. By this time, I was coaching people on keto alongside my boyfriend, who had been a longtime keto specialist, and I felt like I had to walk the walk. I believed keto was "better," even though it clearly wasn't better for *me.* Most of our clients were getting excellent results and raved about how much they loved keto, so I kept thinking I was doing something wrong and just needed to find my "keto sweet spot."

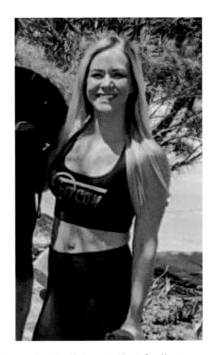

As that year came to a close, I started to venture into eating some carbs again. I had done some DNA and gut testing, and every test I took resulted in the recommendation that I eat a diet rich in carbohydrates.

Intuitively, I had known that was what I needed to do all along. I knew my body felt *way* better when I ate healthy carbs. These test results were just the pushes I needed to listen to that feeling. Sadly, I thought I needed an external source to tell me what felt right for me, but I did.

After just a few months of reintroducing carbs, I got another DEXA scan. My body fat had dropped to 14 percent, and I was up over 2 pounds of muscle mass.

Six months later, I got another scan. I was now at 12.8 percent body fat and up 2 more pounds of muscle mass. Eleven months into bringing carbs back in, I was at 13 percent body fat and up 4 *more* pounds of muscle mass.

So, fifteen months after getting off keto, I had gained 8 pounds of muscle and lost 7 pounds of fat, with no changes to my training routine.

SCAN FROM DEXA BODY

I also had blood work done in the heart of my keto phase and then again three years after I began regularly eating carbohydrates again. My blood panels had improved on almost every biomarker after reintroducing carbohydrates.

Tara Garrison   **Measured: 07/31/2019**

Age: 36.8   Birth Date:
Gender: Female   Height: 67.0 in.

SUMMARY LEVEL RESULTS

Total Body Composition

Measured Date	Total Body Fat	Total Mass (lbs)	Fat Tissue (lbs)	Lean Tissue (lbs)	Bone Mineral Content (BMC)
07/31/2019	15.1%	149.9 lbs	21.80 lbs	122.25 lbs	5.85 lbs
01/10/2019	13.0%	149.3 lbs	18.57 lbs	124.77 lbs	5.97 lbs
08/06/2018	12.8%	144.2 lbs	17.64 lbs	120.55 lbs	6.00 lbs
02/27/2018	14.2%	144.5 lbs	19.65 lbs	118.85 lbs	6.02 lbs
09/19/2017	18.1%	148.4 lbs	25.68 lbs	116.58 lbs	6.12 lbs
05/23/2017	17.1%	151.9 lbs	25.00 lbs	120.85 lbs	6.04 lbs
05/01/2017	17.0%	154.3 lbs	25.20 lbs	123.05 lbs	6.09 lbs
01/05/2017	11.3%	143.7 lbs	15.55 lbs	122.14 lbs	5.97 lbs

Total Body Tissue Quantitation

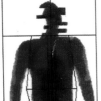

Recommended Body Fat %

This table provides target body fat percentages based on empirical DEXA scan results. It is meant to provide general guidance for individuals, and to help set goals. (Sample Size n=754)

WOMEN
(Essential Fat 10-13%)

Age	0 - 20th Percentile (Athlete)	20th - 40th Percentile (Fitness)	40th - 60th Percentile (Average)	> 60th Percentile (Above Avg)
20-29	< 24%	24% - 28%	28% - 32%	> 32%
30-39	< 26%	26% - 30%	30% - 34%	> 34%
40-49	< 27%	27% - 31%	31% - 35%	> 35%
50-59	< 29%	29% - 33%	33% - 37%	> 38%
>60	< 30%	30% - 34%	34% - 39%	> 39%

MEN
(Essential Fat 5-7%)

Age	0 - 20th Percentile (Athlete)	20th - 40th Percentile (Fitness)	40th - 60th Percentile (Average)	> 60th Percentile (Above Avg)
20-29	< 15%	15% - 18%	18% - 23%	> 23%
30-39	< 16%	16% - 21%	21% - 25%	> 25%
40-49	< 18%	18% - 24%	24% - 27%	> 27%
50-59	< 19%	19% - 25%	25% - 28%	> 28%
> 60	< 24%	24% - 27%	27% - 32%	> 32%

Regional Composition

The table below divides your body into 5 key regions and provides the composition breakdown for each. Dexa Body will track these regions over time to chart individual progress.

Region	Total Region Fat %	Total Mass (lbs)	Fat Tissue (lbs)	Lean Tissue (lbs)	Bone Mineral Content (BMC)
Arms	17.3%	17.2 lbs	2.99 lbs	13.53 lbs	0.73 lbs
Legs	19.4%	55.0 lbs	10.66 lbs	42.13 lbs	2.18 lbs
Trunk	9.4%	68.3 lbs	6.45 lbs	59.99 lbs	1.84 lbs
Android	7.3%	9.6 lbs	0.70 lbs	8.82 lbs	0.10 lbs
Gynoid	16.9%	23.7 lbs	4.00 lbs	19.12 lbs	0.58 lbs

WHILE I WAS ON KETO:	AFTER A FEW YEARS OF BRINGING CARBOHYDRATES BACK IN:
My total cholesterol was 268 (over 240 is conventionally considered high risk).	My total cholesterol was 190 (lower and within the normal range).
My LDL (traditionally considered "bad" cholesterol) was 149 (over 130 is conventionally considered high risk).	My LDL was 110 (lower and within the normal range).
My HDL ("good" cholesterol) was 104 (over 60 is conventionally considered low risk).	My HDL was 67 (significantly lower but still within the normal range).
My triglycerides were 54 (under 150 is considered low risk).	My triglycerides were 50 (lower and within the normal range).
My non-HDL cholesterol (all "less healthy" cholesterol) was 164 (over 160 is considered high risk).	My non-HDL cholesterol was 123 (lower and within the normal range).
My thyroid panels were all normal, except my total T3 was 73 (80 to 81 is considered low risk).	My total T3 shot up to 114 (higher and within the normal range).
My omega-3 index was 3.5 (over 3.2 is considered low risk).	My omega-3 index was 1.3 (significantly lower and high risk).*
My omega-6:omega-3 ratio was 10.3 (between 5.2 and 12.9 is considered low risk).	My omega-6:omega-3 ratio was 10.7 (slightly higher but still within the normal range).
My EPA:arachidonic acid ratio was 0.1 (under 0.2 is considered high risk).	My EPA:AA ratio was 0.1 (no change; high risk).
My red blood cell count was 5.25 (over 5.2 is considered high risk).	My red blood cell count was 4.54 (lower and within the normal range).

*Omega-3 index was the only significant negative change after the reintroduction of carbs. It could be due to the fact that I was inconsistent with taking omega-3 supplements for some time before this blood test, whereas I'd been taking them consistently while on keto.

In regard to cholesterol, the conversation is changing, and there is some emerging evidence that high cholesterol is not as closely associated with cardiovascular disease as was once thought. For example, new research is indicating that low-density lipoprotein (LDL), which has historically been considered a risk factor for atherosclerosis when elevated, may not be the whole story. It appears that the number of small particles within a person's LDL may be the truer indicator of heart disease risk, not LDL itself.[1] But even the leading researchers in this area admit that they don't know for sure. (My small-particle-size LDL was also elevated during my keto phase.)

Please note that this is just my experience with keto. Many, many people have the reverse experience. Their body composition improves on keto, and their blood panels improve as well. A person's response to keto is highly individual. But I want to get the point across that while it's great to lay some of the metabolic groundwork by doing a phase of keto in terms of training your body to run on fat for fuel, it's not an optimal long-term solution for everyone, including me.

Overall, my health improved significantly after I brought carbs back in. Unfortunately, I don't have blood labs from before starting keto for comparison.

I think it's significant that I didn't track my food intake during either phase, so caloric restriction didn't play a factor in my results. In terms of caloric intake, I was eating intuitively—eating only when hungry and stopping when full—during both my keto phase and after reintroducing carbs. While eating keto, I tracked carbs in my mind and checked my blood ketone levels often to make sure I was staying in ketosis. But I never tracked calories or macros. This was purely the result of what happened when I ate keto and what happened when I reincorporated healthy whole-food carbohydrates.

So, while I had more favorable outcomes across the board when eating healthy carbohydrates, I am grateful for the positive impact of my keto phase—I had better mental clarity, did not experience afternoon dips in energy, and felt much better in the absence of incoming food. "Hanger" was a thing of the past. I could perform in the gym whether I had eaten or not, and I could go many hours without eating and feel absolutely fine. Fasting, which I do occasionally for the health benefits described in Chapter 4, became so much easier. By going keto, I trained my body well to run on its own fat stores for energy.

That is why I still recommend a keto phase for most people. It's like a metabolic boot camp where you train your metabolism to run at full capacity. The amazing thing I noticed after bringing carbs back in was that I maintained all these benefits. I could still go long periods without feeling hungry or hangry, fasted like a champ, performed extremely well while fasted in the gym, and felt mentally amazing with no afternoon dips in energy, just like when I was in ketosis. I had benefited from some amazing metabolic adaptations from keto, and I was now bringing those advantages with me, even when eating carbohydrates again.

AFTER KETO

While I was going through this experience, the internet and social media were being plastered with messages about keto being "the" optimal way for humans to eat. The general public had caught hold of the message, and the keto frenzy was spreading like wildfire. I was also immersed in the ketogenic professional community. While I agreed with much of what my colleagues were saying, I felt there was more to the story that wasn't being shared. I knew I needed to speak up. I had to talk about my experience, share my knowledge, and do what my gut was not-so-gently nudging me to do.

It was actually very scary to speak my truth. Crazy, right? It kind of felt like I was leaving a cult or going against my religion. I had, by then, become friends with many leaders in the keto industry. All of a sudden, I was going to be saying something different from what all of my peers—my community of like-minded people—had been saying. How would they take it? How much heat was I going to get? Was I going to become an outcast?

I'll never forget the day I posted this picture of a sweet potato on my plate on Instagram. I thought I would surely be rejected from the keto community forever. My career as a keto specialist would be over.

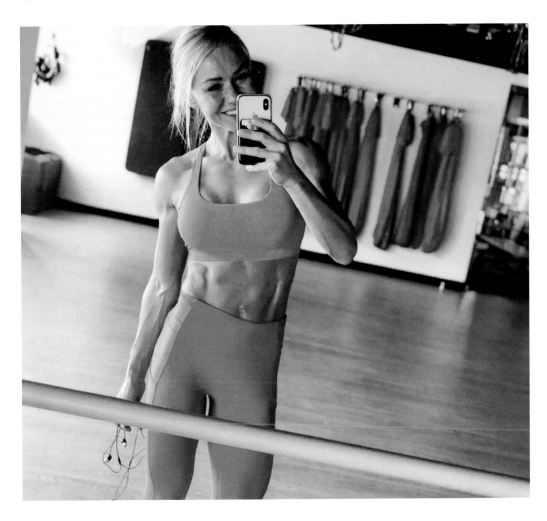

There was not a single other keto specialist at that time—none that I knew of, anyway—speaking in favor of carbohydrates *at all.* But I felt I had to do it. So I started to share how much better I was feeling and looking after bringing carbs back in.

Right around that time, I attended KetoCon in Austin, Texas. This was 2018, when keto was at its pinnacle. Back then, to even suggest to that tribe that carbs were healthy was blasphemy. Yet here I was, walking around at a ketogenic conference, a living testament that carbs can be good for you and that keto isn't the be-all and end-all for all humans. It was a very interesting position to be in. I knew the benefits of a ketogenic diet, and I knew keto was an incredible tool for so many of my clients and others I had met. But I really disliked the dogmatic zeal around it that I was seeing. Carbs were made out to be the enemy when they clearly weren't for me or, as research shows, millions of others.

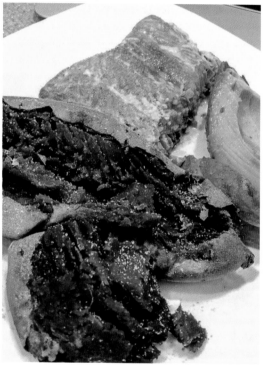

At the conference, I was working a booth for my friend Drew Manning, who had sold hundreds of thousands of copies of his keto program. Some of the people I met there knew who I was from social media, and what happened next felt like divine intervention—like the universe was telling me to speak up.

Three different women came up to me at the booth, practically begging for help. Their stories were almost identical: "I've been keto for _____ years, and I can't lose weight. I've tried everything—more fat, less fat, more protein, less protein, more calories, fewer calories, more lifting, not lifting at all, different types of exercise, fasting, not fasting.... What gives?! Why can't I lose weight?"

I asked all three of them, "Have you tried bringing carbs back in?"

They all looked at me like deer in headlights, utterly shocked that I would ask such a question.

"REALLY?" they responded.

When I got home, I couldn't stop thinking about the conversations I'd had. I felt like people were being indoctrinated instead of being given food for thought. They were being brainwashed, convinced, sold. They were being made to feel wrong if keto wasn't delivering its promised miracles. It really started to bug me.

I thought about how many of my keto influencer friends sometimes cycled carbs in. I had been to lunches and dinners with these friends and noticed that while they were generally keto, they would occasionally eat sweet potato fries or potatoes or sweet potatoes at home after a workout. They knew that their bodies could handle an occasional "carb-up," that it would likely boost their muscle glycogen for athletic performance the next day, and that they would return to ketosis quickly since they weren't consuming a ton of carbs.

At that time, however, this was not what the general public was hearing. All they were hearing in the online keto community was they should be doing 100 percent keto, 100 percent of the time. The message was that carbs were bad, and if you were "in the know," you knew it. Even cyclical keto or targeted keto (where carbs are strategically incorporated into a ketogenic diet) were barely mentioned back then; most people didn't even know what those approaches were. (See Chapter 4 for more on this approach.)

Don't get me wrong; I was still a fan of keto. For many of my clients, it was a powerful tool to enhance their health—a miraculous intervention. As mentioned earlier, I loved what it had done for my own mental state and my ability to go long periods of time without food and feel great.

But long term? Keto was not the answer for me, and it wasn't the answer for some of my clients, either. I had many clients who didn't get the results they wanted on keto, and when they switched to low to moderate carbs, everything got better.

I had also learned that for many people, keto worked...until it didn't. Once keto had done its job of reducing inflammation, restoring insulin sensitivity, balancing hormones, and so on, it had diminishing returns. Many times, people started gaining weight or not feeling as great as they once had.

I became concerned about the disordered eating patterns I was seeing in many ketogenic dieters, too. They had developed an extreme fear of carbohydrates and felt terrible guilt when they would inevitably "cave" and eat them. Those caving moments usually led to all-out carbohydrate binges, and restrict-and-binge cycles ensued. If not that, then they threw the towel in altogether and went back to the standard American diet full of all their old favorite processed foods. They developed black-and-white thinking, as though the only way to be healthy was to be keto. They were either

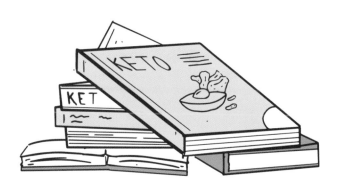

all in or all out; there was no middle ground in which they simply enjoyed healthy carbohydrates in moderation.

So there I was, smack dab in the middle of the keto community, anything but a keto zealot.

I loved the results my clients were getting from doing keto for a period of time and then bringing healthy carbs back in. They developed amazing appetite regulation, high energy levels, and a healthy relationship with all three macronutrients.

I started to teach the message "Do keto. Not forever." I encouraged people to do a phase of keto, see how they felt, train their metabolism to run on fat for fuel and easily tap into their fat stores, and then experiment with bringing carbs back in and return to balance.

Since then, I've coached hundreds of people one-on-one and in my Keto In & Out program, and I've seen the beauty of this process over and over again. Once my clients reintroduce healthy carbohydrates after a keto phase, they are able to maintain their fit lifestyle and get the body composition results they're after—all without developing a restrictive mindset around food.

So I'm bringing you this book to teach my "Do keto. Not forever." approach at a deeper level. I'm excited to share with you the reasons I still support doing a phase of keto and why, when, and how to bring healthy carbohydrates back in for a sustainable lifestyle and optimal body composition.

REFERENCES

1. Ronald M. Krauss, "All Low-Density Lipoprotein Particles Are Not Created Equal," *Arteriosclerosis, Thrombosis, and Vascular Biology* 34, no. 5 (2014): 959–61, https://doi.org/10.1161/ATVBAHA.114.303458.

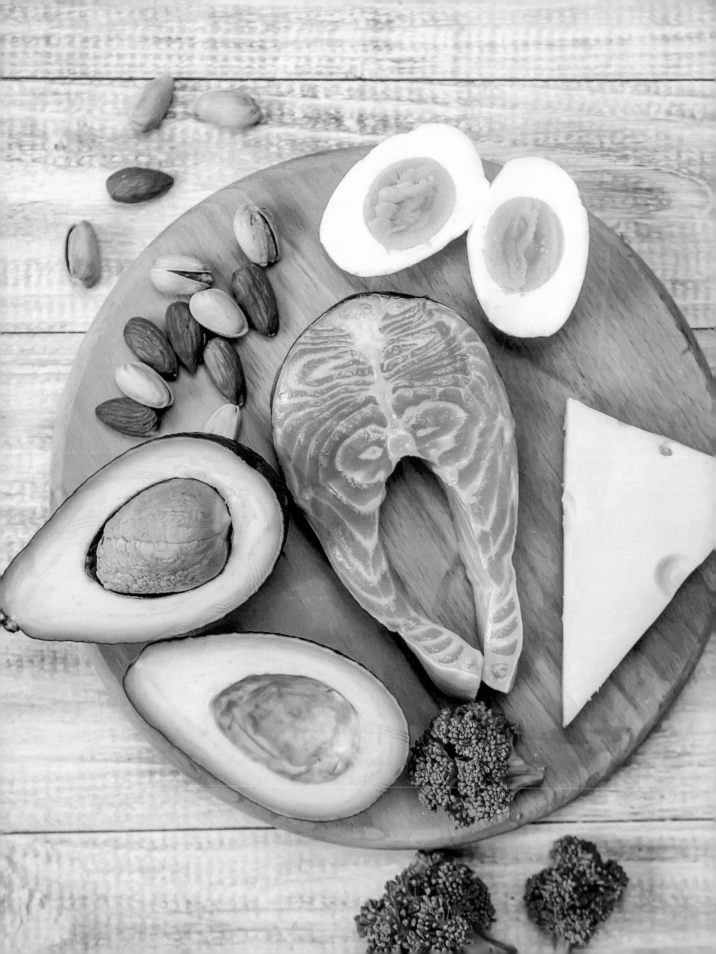

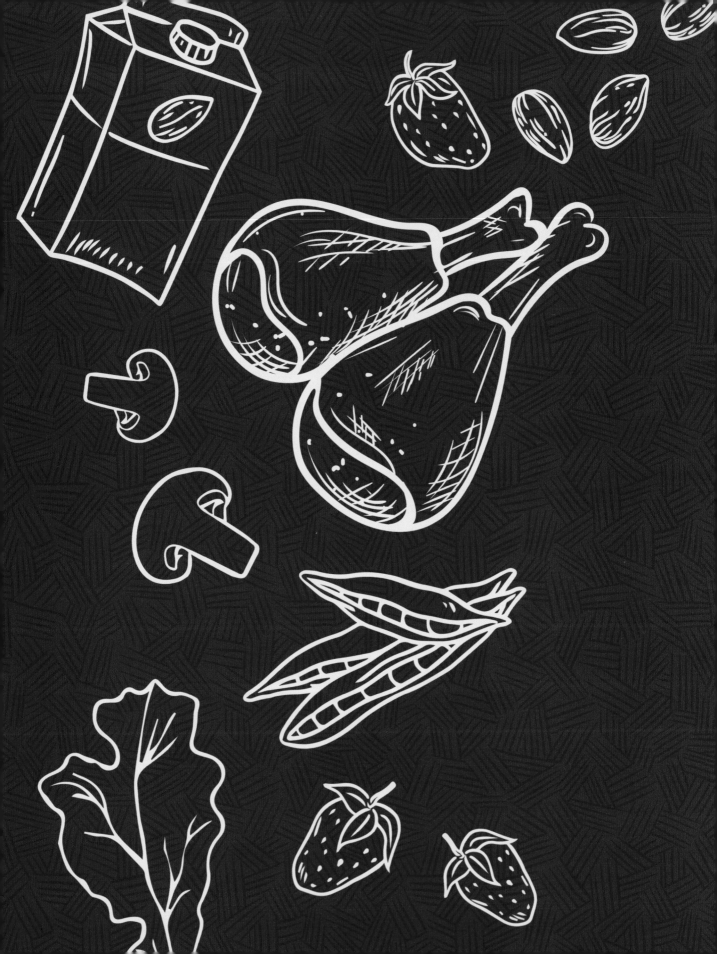

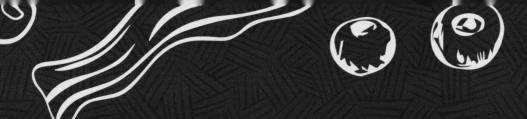

CHAPTER 1

WHY KETO IS A SMART MOVE

There are a lot of strong opinions when it comes to keto, both for and against the diet. Some people are keto enthusiasts, while others are skeptical.

The keto enthusiasts are confident that they have discovered *the* optimal form of human nutrition. They often make it their mission in life to help other people feel as good as they do on keto. Some of these enthusiasts are nutritionists, doctors, health coaches, and researchers. Others are people who have seen life-changing improvements in their health from keto and just want to share the science, research, and anecdotal stories that support their beliefs and experiences. They feel better, they've seen other people feel better, and they believe they can help everyone else feel better, too...if they will just do keto.

Then we have the keto skeptics. Many of them are also nutritionists, doctors, and researchers who recognize the value of keto but argue that it's an unnecessary and unsustainable intervention for most of the population. They are concerned about potential risk factors that keto advocates tend to downplay. Over and over I have seen keto advocates snub their noses at these professionals, claiming that they are "behind the times" or just don't get it.

The reality, though, is that many of them *do* get it. They understand keto and why people like it. And they usually agree that keto can be helpful for certain conditions, such as high inflammation, obesity, metabolic syndrome, type 2 diabetes, and neurological disorders. However, they also have their eyes wide open about the downsides. They know that keto isn't the only way to help with these issues, and they aren't convinced that dramatically reducing consumption of an entire macronutrient is going to serve people overall and in their long-term health.

I can't even tell you how interesting it has been to sit back and consider both sides objectively while actively coaching people in and out of the keto diet.

I like to keep an open mind. Since not one person on the planet fully understands the human body, I believe health professionals have an obligation to remain open-minded.

I have clients who *thrive* on keto and sing my praises for saving their lives. Keto is the only thing that has ever worked for them; their entire lives are better because of keto.

And I have clients for whom keto didn't work. These clients didn't enjoy the experience of being on keto and didn't get the results they wanted, no matter how much we optimized and tweaked the diet. Pretty much all of them got excited in the beginning when they dropped 5 to 10 pounds (the first half of which was mostly water weight), and they felt better for a time—most likely from a reduction in inflammation and from cutting sugar and many processed foods out of their diets. But after that? Diminishing returns. Their body composition just wouldn't move in the right direction, their exercise performance dropped, and they didn't feel as good. They almost always felt better and got results when we brought carbohydrates back in.

Here is what I've learned: *both groups are right.* Keto works when nothing else does; it saves lives. At the same time, keto doesn't work. It isn't the ticket for everyone. It depends on the individual.

In this chapter, I will discuss why keto works—and I'm not just talking about fat loss. Perhaps the biggest reason people oppose keto is that they are looking at it as a weight-loss diet. While viewing keto just as a super-restrictive, unsustainable, extreme weight-loss tactic, they are entirely missing the boat on what the diet is supposed to do: heal.

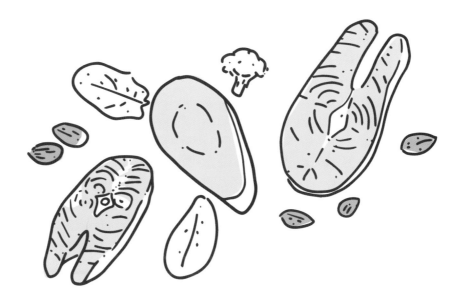

THE THERAPEUTIC
ORIGINS OF KETO

The ketogenic diet doesn't have its origins in weight loss; it entered the medical scene as a healing tool. Fat loss was simply a surprise side effect.

Keto was used as a healing modality for epilepsy starting in the early 1900s. It continues to be used today as a healing strategy for a wide variety of conditions, including migraines, traumatic brain injury, Alzheimer's, Parkinson's disease, sleep disorders, brain cancer, autism, ADHD, multiple sclerosis, polycystic ovarian syndrome, diabetes, and metabolic syndrome.

In my practice, I have helped hypothyroid clients reduce or stop thyroid medication by taking them through a phase of the ketogenic diet and then reintroducing carbohydrates. I believe the reduction in gut inflammation, the anti-inflammatory nature of ketone bodies, and the improvement in blood sugar regulation all helped. Many of these clients were also over-exercisers, which likely contributed to elevated cortisol and blood sugar, both of which lead to weight gain and inflammation. As a result, we reduced the amount of exercise they did, went through a phase of keto, and took a holistic/spiritual healing approach at the same time.

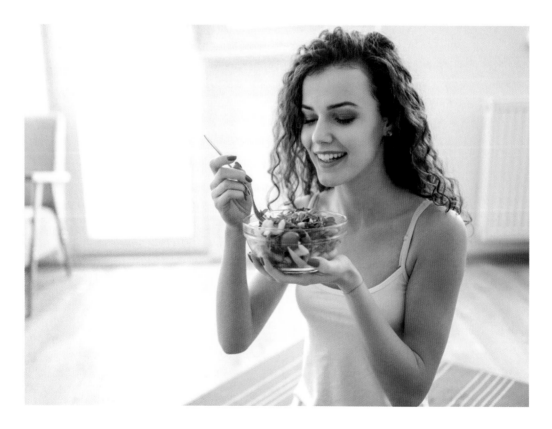

HOW READY ACCESS TO FOOD WORKS AGAINST OUR BIOLOGY

What if you don't have any major health issues? Should you even bother with keto? Especially if you love carbs?

For many of us, getting rid of carbs sounds terrible! I feel you. I love carbs, too. But I believe going through a phase of the ketogenic diet will do just about everyone a major metabolic favor. Why? Because keto is an amazing biohack that trains our bodies to do what they're naturally supposed to do on a regular basis but do not do because of the modern, food-abundant world so many of us live in.

Going into a state of ketosis is as natural as it gets. Our bodies were designed to do this! Many people believe you have to eat a high-fat ketogenic diet to enter ketosis, but you actually don't have to eat any fat at all. In fact, fasting—eating nothing—is the quickest way to get into ketosis. Human beings evolved on periods of fasting, ranging from several hours to several days, purely from a lack of food being available to them in the wild. And we get some fantastic health benefits when we allow our bodies to go into that fasted state, which I'll describe later in this book. But how often do we actually enter that state in our food-abundant world? When was the last time you went eighteen to twenty-four hours without eating?

We have a big problem collectively as human beings. We rarely go into ketosis anymore because for the first time in human history—really just in the last 100 years in most areas of the world—not only do many of us have virtually unlimited access to food, but we also barely have to move.

This is a *huge* problem for human health.

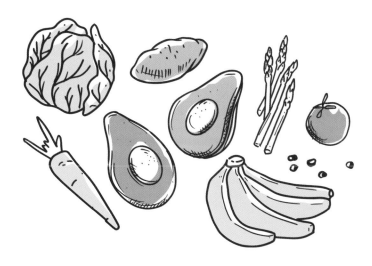

If we lived in nature and had to hunt, gather, or grow our food, we would be moving so much more and eating so much less! We just wouldn't have the option of stuffing our faces with food anytime we felt like it. We wouldn't have food available to us every time we got the least bit hungry. We would be going in and out of ketosis *all the time* because ketogenesis occurs any time we run out of carbohydrates to fuel our bodies. We would enter that ketogenic state easily because our bodies would be used to it. And every time we did, a lot of amazing metabolic adaptations, such as optimized insulin levels, the release of growth hormone, cellular repair, and gene expression that protects against disease, would occur.

In today's world, that's just not likely to happen. Why would we sit there uncomfortably hungry when nearly every food we could ever want is an arm's length away? You want grapes from Mexico? Pineapples from Hawaii? No problem. Drive down the street to the grocery store and grab some. Craving donuts? They can be all yours in less than ten minutes for a buck apiece. Chocolate? Chips? Crackers? You probably already have some in the pantry. Burger and fries? You don't even have to get out of your car! Or shoot, just get it delivered!

Never before have human beings had access to so much food, and it's causing a health crisis. Here's a snapshot:

- As of 2020, 42.4 percent of Americans are obese.[1]

- Approximately 88 million American adults—more than one in three people—have prediabetes. However, it's estimated that 84 percent of them aren't aware that they have it.[2]

- More than 34 million Americans—that's over 10 percent of the population—have type 2 diabetes.[3]

This is because, in a world of food abundance dominated by hyperpalatable, calorically dense processed foods, we are at a face-off between our biology and our environment.

"In a world of food abundance and hyperpalatable, calorically dense processed foods, we are at a face-off between our biology and our environment."

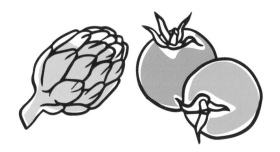

Biologically, our bodies want us to store fat. It's a survival mechanism. That biological drive to eat to excess when food was available served our ancestors well when they were starving in the wild. But now? For most of us, food is rarely scarce. But our bodies don't know that.

On top of wanting to store fat, our bodies don't want to use up their fat stores unless they have to. Again, this is a survival mechanism. In an effort to conserve fat in case of a future famine, when our bodies sense they are getting low on energy from incoming food, they release chemicals that encourage us to eat instead of tapping into the energy we already have stored in the form of fat. So we feel hungry even though we have plenty of energy stored in our bodies.

And hunger is not exactly a comfortable feeling. Since no one loves feeling uncomfortable, what happens? At the slightest sign of hunger, we eat whatever sounds good to us—the peanut M&Ms in a coworker's candy jar, the grilled cheese left on our kids' plates, or a bag of chips lying around in the kitchen. And in so doing, we never allow our bodies to tap into the energy we've already got: our fat stores.

The worst part? As this cycle repeats itself, we become more and more dependent on food for energy. Our bodies actually become convinced that they need incoming food constantly even though they have plenty of energy stashed away. They become spoiled—like a child who lives in a house full of toys but still constantly wants a new one. And the more the parent obliges, the more fervent those demands become.

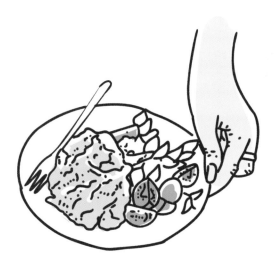

TRAINING OUR BODIES TO RUN ON STORED FAT

This is where keto comes in. This is how we train our bodies to become extremely good at using up the fat they already have. This is how we train our bodies to effortlessly transition into burning their own fat for fuel without having a temper tantrum. (Anyone who has ever been hangry knows what I'm talking about.) This is something we can get better at.

The "keto flu" is a wake-up call that we are generally pretty bad at this transition! And it doesn't have to be that way. We can experience physical hunger but still feel great from an energy standpoint; we just have to train our bodies to do it. And doing a phase of the ketogenic diet is a very effective way to accomplish that goal.

When we put our bodies in a state of ketosis for an extended time—I recommend at least four weeks—we train them to run on fat, whether it's fat from food or our own body fat. This is the training our bodies need. On the flip side, every time we fail to let our bodies learn what to do in the absence of food, we are training them to become dependent on incoming glucose for energy. That's why, if you haven't made an effort to fat-adapt your body, you feel fatigued and foggy-brained when you go a long time without eating. It doesn't have to be like that.

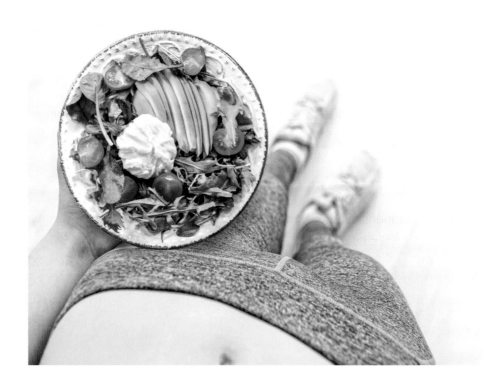

Most people don't even realize that they don't have to feel this way. They think fatigue and brain fog are normal. These feelings are typical, but they are not normal! And they're definitely not necessary. You don't have to feel different from an energy standpoint just because you're hungry. You don't have to feel lethargic in the midafternoon. You don't have to feel agitated if you go a while without food. You don't have to go into panic mode (which usually leads to poor food choices) when it has been several hours since your last meal. You don't have to feel lightheaded, weak, tired, or cranky when you're hungry. Keto can help you overcome that.

If any of this sounds like you, I highly recommend trying a phase of keto to help you overcome it. Train your body on what to do when your blood sugar starts to drop.

Let me share a story about this.

My mother was diagnosed with type 2 diabetes when I was in high school. Now, as a health professional, I can see all the warning signs that were present in the years leading up to that diagnosis. Driving home from church on Sundays, she would always say she had to get something to eat; she just couldn't make the drive home without eating. She would show us how her hands trembled, saying she felt like she was going to pass out. She thought she had hypoglycemia.

One time, my mom had bought a box of Twinkies, and I couldn't wait to have one when I got home from school. When I looked for it, it was nowhere to be found. I asked her where the Twinkies were, and she giggled guiltily, saying, "I ate them all."

I remember saying incredulously, "You ate an *entire box* of Twinkies?!" We laughed, and afterward I would tease her about it. But now that I understand what was really happening, I can see that it was anything but funny. And it wasn't really her fault. She just didn't understand what was happening inside her body. My mom was experiencing, in the extreme, what I've been describing here:

1. You eat hyperpalatable processed foods that are high in carbohydrates with little to no fiber to slow down your blood sugar response.

2. Your blood sugar spikes and then falls.

3. When your blood sugar starts to get low, you feel weak, shaky, and irritable.

4. Instead of getting past that moment and allowing your body to transition into fat-burning mode in order to provide you with energy (like you would do if you lived in the wild and had no other choice), you eat again. Why not? You've got plenty of snacks around. Why sit there and feel uncomfortable if you don't have to?

And this is what happens over and over, year after year, causing you to gain body fat and gradually increasing your blood sugar levels. The reason is that many of the times you're eating, it's not about hunger; it's about blood sugar! You consume all these extra calories in an attempt to regulate your blood sugar when what you really need to do is *not consume any calories at all*—or at least not in the form of carbohydrates—in order to train your body to become better at regulating your blood sugar on its own. This cycle is the beginning of insulin resistance and eventually type 2 diabetes.

Incredible adaptations happen in our bodies when we go without food. But we can achieve similar adaptations while still eating food by following a ketogenic diet. It's an incredible hack in our modern, food-abundant world that allows us to use the full capacity of our metabolism.

Keto makes fat loss easier, especially if you have high blood sugar. If you take someone who has prediabetes or is obese with poor blood sugar regulation and just tell them to restrict calories, they won't succeed; their hunger will get the best of them. Keto is a bridge. It allows a person to eat food, get nice and full, and break free from the chronic hunger associated with blood sugar ups and downs. They will finally feel like they can do it. This will allow them to achieve the metabolic adaptations in their bodies necessary to pave the way for them to more easily restrict calories while eating all three macronutrients in the future. Keto is a metabolic fixer, and a powerful one.

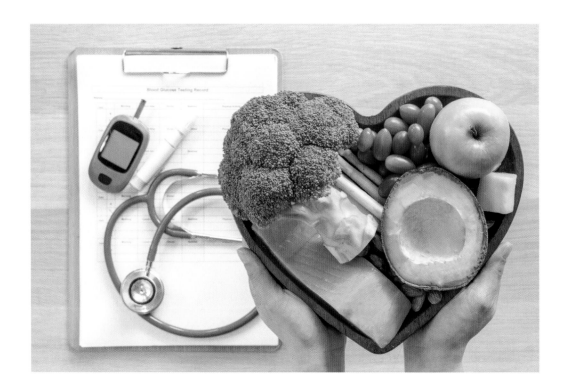

SCIENCE-BACKED BENEFITS OF THE KETOGENIC DIET

As a keto diet specialist who frequently attends ketogenic conferences where doctors and researchers discuss the latest reports on the topic, I would love to share with you some of the science-backed benefits of the keto diet.

Keto isn't a silly fad diet. In fact, if you attended some of these conferences, you'd see that most of the people there didn't get into keto for weight loss. They're using it to heal or prevent metabolic diseases that they're currently experiencing, or that run in their families. Many of them use it as a life optimization tool because they have experienced the mental clarity that often comes with the diet. Many are longevity geeks who just want to live a long time and enjoy a high quality of life.

My favorite of these events is the Metabolic Health Summit. I can pretty much guarantee that if you are a keto skeptic and you attend that conference, you will no longer look at keto as a fad diet. I would be shocked if you didn't attempt keto yourself after hearing the research findings presented at this summit.

So let's dig into those.

- **Keto can improve cognitive function.** Studies show that people with mild to moderate neurocognitive impairment experience improvement in executive function (working memory, flexible thinking, self-control) and speed of processing when on a ketogenic diet.[4]

- **Keto can reduce inflammation.** Your mitochondria generate energy in the form of adenosine triphosphate (ATP) to fuel your cells. That process creates free radicals, also known as reactive oxygen species, as a by-product. Free radicals are unstable atoms that can damage cells, causing illness as we age. Obviously, since we are producing ATP every second of our lives, our bodies are prepared for this; they minimize the damage by creating endogenous (meaning "made within the body") antioxidants like glutathione. But if the free radical load becomes too great, it causes us to age prematurely and increases our risk of stroke and neurodegeneration. Ketones directly inhibit inflammation and oxidative stress by enhancing the breakdown of free radicals and increasing the activity of our innate antioxidant system.[5]

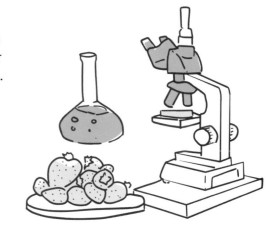

- **Keto can decrease appetite, making fat loss easier.** A study that compared a ketogenic diet and a low-fat diet found that the participants in the ketogenic group experienced less hunger than those in the low-fat group.[6]

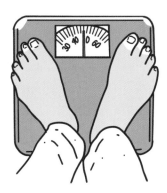

- **Keto can lower triglycerides.** Studies on overweight and obese subjects have found that a keto diet can drastically lower triglycerides, which are one of the biggest contributors to cardiovascular problems.[7]

- **Keto can increase good cholesterol.** One of the easiest ways to increase HDL, your "good cholesterol," is to eat healthy fats. Keto definitely helps with this effort.[8]

- **Keto can lower blood sugar and insulin levels.** Dropping carbs has led to impressive results for people with type 2 diabetes and insulin resistance. In one study of patients with type 2 diabetes and obesity, 95 percent eliminated their glucose-lowering medication within six months of starting a low-carbohydrate diet.[9]

- **Keto can preserve existing neurons and stimulate the production of new, healthy ones.**[10]

- **Keto can help the body kill off old, damaged cells and create new, healthy ones.**[11]

- **Keto can help heal and protect against neurodegenerative diseases.** For people with neurological disorders such as epilepsy, Parkinson's disease, Alzheimer's, dementia, or migraines, keto may be a life-changing healing modality.[12]

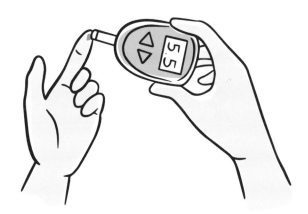

- **Keto can promote healing for autoimmune disease, polycystic ovarian syndrome (PCOS), some types of cancer, and metabolic syndrome.** While research on keto and autoimmune disease is limited, a large amount of anecdotal evidence points to the promise of keto's impact on reducing inflammation and consequently autoimmune symptoms. In research, implementing a ketogenic diet has been shown to reduce symptoms of PCOS, the most common endocrine disorder for women of childbearing age. Rodent studies and small human studies have also shown benefits of the ketogenic diet in regard to cancer, particularly glioblastoma (an aggressive type of brain cancer), prostate, breast, liver, and stomach cancers. Scientists believe that these benefits are due not only to the starving of the tumors, which feed on sugar, but also to the fact that keto changes gene expression, which in turn changes the way cells behave. Nutritional ketosis has been found to serve as a treatment for metabolic syndrome by improving metabolic and inflammatory markers, including HbA1c, CRP, fasting insulin, and glucose levels, as well as aiding in weight loss, decreasing hunger, and increasing satiety.[13]

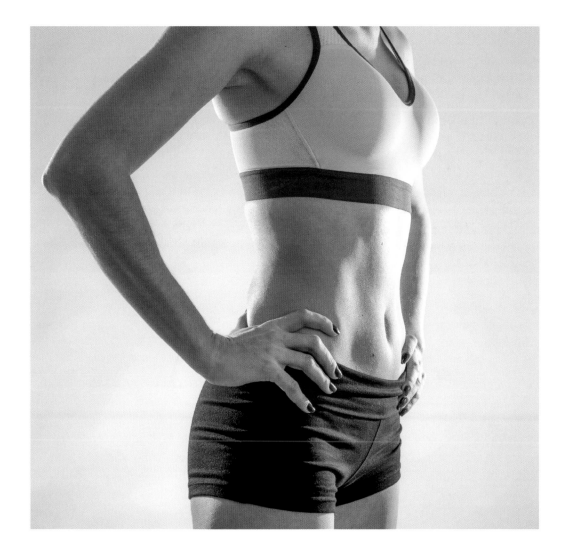

As you can see, keto is not just a fad diet for people who want to lose weight. It's one of the most researched diets there is. It deserves a seat at the table when it comes to improving human health. In addition to all of these therapeutic applications, keto is an extremely powerful tool to quickly and effectively swing the metabolic pendulum back to a healthy place. It is a metabolic enhancer that allows people to feel their best without needing a constant influx of carbohydrates.

My favorite aspect of the ketogenic diet is its powerful ability to regulate blood sugar. It makes fat loss so much easier for people with high blood sugar, which is becoming incredibly common. To someone with high blood sugar, the idea of eating at a calorie deficit or forgoing sugar can seem nearly impossible. When their blood sugar drops after a carbohydrate-rich meal, their cravings for more carbs can be so intense that even the most strong-willed will be unable to resist. They haven't yet trained their bodies on what to do when they run out of incoming glucose. Instead of knowing they can tap into stored fat for fuel, their bodies freak out, thinking they need energy *stat,* and off they rush to the pantry or a fast-food restaurant. Keto provides a temporary space in which blood sugar levels remain stable, so cravings go down. And in this space, people build the metabolic environment that will keep them feeling great with or without a constant supply of incoming glucose.

Keto is extremely effective for healing the metabolic dysfunction created by the low-fat, high-carb recommendations that were prevalent over the past few decades and the industrialization of food, making processed, hyperpalatable, and hypercaloric foods the norm.

Without an abundance of food, would we need extreme dietary interventions like keto? Probably not. Out of sheer force, we would go into and out of ketosis all the time. If all we could find to eat was an animal, we would live off that food source and be in ketosis for who knows how long. If we found a bunch of fruit, we would feast on that and then roll right back into ketosis because food was in short supply. However, since most of us do not willingly go hungry very often, keto is an amazing hack to get the same benefits while still eating certain foods.

I hope I'm getting the point across here that keto helps create metabolic freedom, often referred to as metabolic flexibility. Teaching our bodies how to run well without a constant supply of incoming glucose is *really* healthy. If our bodies know how to do this, we can avoid becoming part of the epidemics of type 2 diabetes, obesity, and metabolic syndrome. We can learn what it feels like to eat according to actual hunger and not to cravings that come as a result of low blood sugar.

So, if you have already done keto, or if perhaps you are following a ketogenic diet right now, you made a smart move. You taught your body how to run well without relying on carbohydrates. If you haven't done keto yet, I highly recommend trying it. Training your body to run on ketones and, therefore, to use the full capacity of its metabolism is one of the best things you can do. The ideal human metabolism doesn't run on only glucose or only ketones; it can use either as a primary fuel source, and it can switch between the two with ease. That's the ideal.

If you haven't gone through a phase of the ketogenic diet, I suggest that you try it for a month, which is the minimum amount of time it typically takes to get the full benefit of a keto phase. By the end of that month, you should have a pretty good idea of how your body feels on keto.

That being said, the period of time I'd recommend for doing keto depends heavily on the individual. If you would like help through my keto program, or to get individual coaching help with keto, you can check my website (taragarrison.com). For now, let's shift gears and talk about why, even though keto is beneficial for most people, I don't think you need to do it forever.

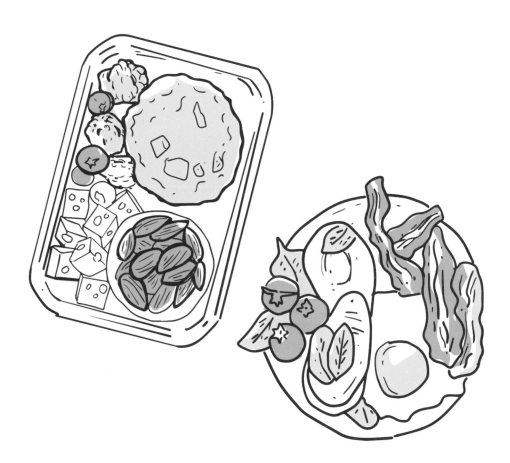

REFERENCES

1. Centers for Disease Control and Prevention, "Prevalence of Obesity and Severe Obesity Among Adults: United States, 2017–2018," NCHS Data Brief no. 360 (2020): 1–8, https://www.cdc.gov/nchs/products/databriefs/db360.htm.

2. Centers for Disease Control and Prevention, "Prediabetes–Your Chance to Prevent Type 2 Diabetes," accessed June 27, 2021, https://www.cdc.gov/diabetes/basics/prediabetes.html.

3. Centers for Disease Control and Prevention, "Type 2 Diabetes," accessed June 27, 2021, https://www.cdc.gov/diabetes/basics/type2.html.

4. Shannon A. Morrison et al., "Cognitive Effects of a Ketogenic Diet on Neurocognitive Impairment in Adults Aging with HIV: A Pilot Study," *Journal of the Association of Nurses in AIDS Care* 31, no. 3 (2020): 312–24, https://doi.org/10.1097/JNC.0000000000000110.

5. Tiffany Greco et al., "Ketogenic Diet Decreases Oxidative Stress and Improves Mitochondrial Respiratory Complex Activity," *Journal of Cerebral Blood Flow and Metabolism* 36, no. 9 (2016): 1603–13, https://doi.org/10.1177/0271678X15610584.

6. F. J. McClernon et al., "The Effects of a Low-Carbohydrate Ketogenic Diet and a Low-Fat Diet on Mood, Hunger, and Other Self-Reported Symptoms," *Obesity* 15, no. 1 (2007): 182–7, https://doi.org/10.1038/oby.2007.516.

7. Richard J. Wood et al., "Carbohydrate Restriction Alters Lipoprotein Metabolism by Modifying VLDL, LDL, and HDL Subfraction Distribution and Size in Overweight Men," *Journal of Nutrition* 136, no. 2 (2006): 384–9, https://doi.org/10.1093/jn/136.2.384.

8. Ronald P. Mensink et al., "Effects of Dietary Fatty Acids and Carbohydrates on the Ratio of Serum Total to HDL Cholesterol and on Serum Lipids and Apolipoproteins: A Meta-Analysis of 60 Controlled Trials," *American Journal of Clinical Nutrition* 77, no. 5 (2003): 1146–55, https://doi.org/10.1093/ajcn/77.5.1146.

9. Eric C. Westman et al., "The Effect of a Low-Carbohydrate, Ketogenic Diet Versus a Low-Glycemic Index Diet on Glycemic Control in Type 2 Diabetes Mellitus," *Nutrition & Metabolism* 5, no. 1 (2008), https://doi.org/10.1186/1743-7075-5-36.

10. See note 6 above.

11. Chia-Wei Cheng et al., "Ketone Body Signaling Mediates Intestinal Stem Cell Homeostasis and Adaptation to Diet," *Cell* 178, no. 5 (2019): 1115–31, https://doi.org/10.1016/j.cell.2019.07.048.

12. Dariusz Włodarek, "Role of Ketogenic Diets in Neurodegenerative Diseases (Alzheimer's Disease and Parkinson's Disease)," *Nutrients* 11, no. 1 (2019): 169, https://doi.org/10.3390/nu11010169.

13. Amanda Cabrera-Mulero et al., "Keto Microbiota: A Powerful Contributor to Host Disease Recovery," *Reviews in Endocrine & Metabolic Disorders* 20, no. 4 (2019): 415–25, https://doi.org/10.1007/s11154-019-09518-8; John C. Mavropoulos et al., "The Effects of a Low-Carbohydrate, Ketogenic Diet on the Polycystic Ovary Syndrome: A Pilot Study," *Nutrition & Metabolism* 2 (2005): 35, https://doi.org/10.1186/1743-7075-2-35; Jocelyn Tan-Shalaby, "Ketogenic Diets and Cancer: Emerging Evidence," *Federal Practitioner* 34, Suppl 1 (2017): 37S–42S; Victoria M. Gershuni, Stephanie L. Yan, and Valentina Medici, "Nutritional Ketosis for Weight Management and Reversal of Metabolic Syndrome," *Current Nutrition Reports* 7, no. 3 (2018): 97–106, https://doi.org/10.1007/s13668-018-0235-0.

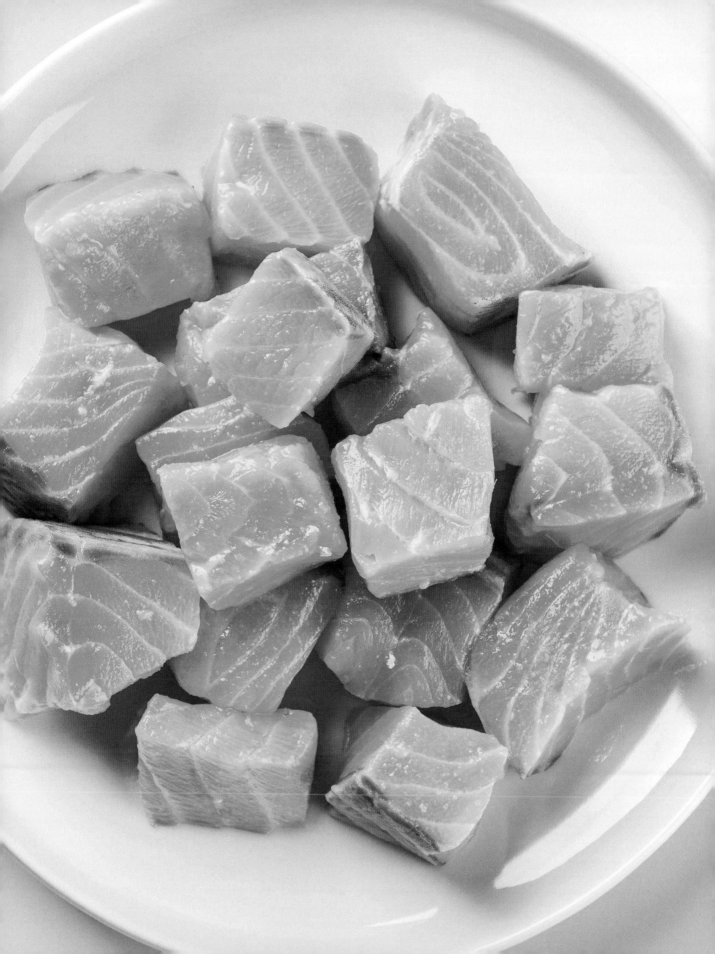

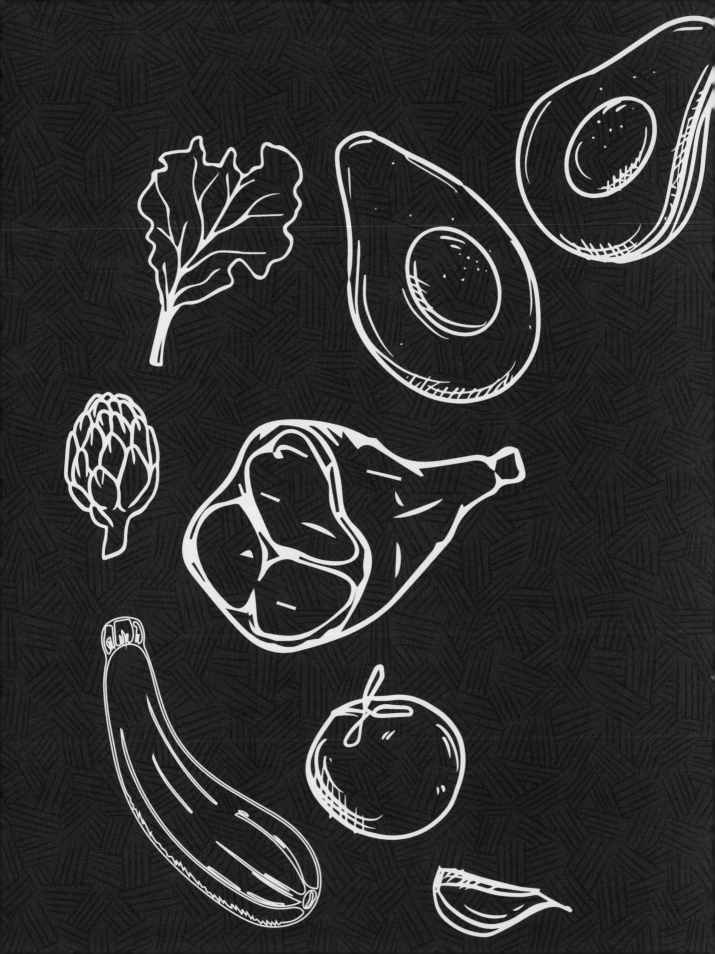

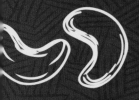

CHAPTER 2

IF KETO IS SO AWESOME, WHY NOT STAY KETO FOREVER?

In the previous chapter, I discussed the many benefits of going through a phase of a ketogenic diet. In this chapter, I'll talk about why I don't advocate being on a ketogenic diet forever.

While a very small percentage of the population may do well on a long-term ketogenic diet, this is unnecessary and likely not optimal for most people. I will discuss the many reasons why in this chapter.

On the simplest, most obvious level, we look to nature. Not only are natural carbohydrates abundantly available to us, but our bodies are designed to run primarily on carbohydrates. We know that human beings have evolved dramatically over at least the last 100,000 years by eating carbohydrates. We have evidence that cooked starch, a source of preformed glucose, greatly increased energy availability to human tissues with high glucose demands, such as the brain, red blood cells, and the developing fetus.[1]

When our metabolisms are functioning correctly, eating carbohydrates is incredibly healthy. Natural sources of carbohydrates are very nutritious; they are chock-full of vitamins, minerals, amino acids, phytonutrients, fiber, and more. Glucose is our bodies' preferred energy source. We can run on ketones, but when we eat fat and carbs, our bodies will run primarily on the carbs! If that doesn't tell us our bodies want carbohydrates, I don't know what does.

So, when we severely restrict carbohydrates, not only are we missing out on so many of the nutrients available to us, but we also increase our risk of adrenal fatigue, higher cortisol, lower serotonin, and other negative consequences that will be discussed later in the chapter.

Once you've trained your body how to easily transition into ketosis, staying keto 100 percent of the time forever is only really necessary in extreme cases, when someone has a medical issue that they are managing therapeutically with a ketogenic diet. The rest of us should be able to eat carbs and feel great, and run on ketones and feel great, easily transitioning between the two metabolic states.

We use keto as a means to get to that place. Keto is the tool, not the destination. For many, it's a life-changing dietary intervention that restores healthy metabolic function. But the goal is to get back to a place where we can eat protein, fat, and carbs again and feel amazing.

Just like keto can correct a lot of things that we miss out on when we are chronically dependent on glucose, we also miss out on some things when we are chronically dependent on ketones—especially in terms of body composition and athletic performance. The right kinds of carbs can actually make improving body composition a lot easier, and there are just certain things we can do better from an athletic standpoint when we eat carbohydrates.

For example, let's compare the following two people.

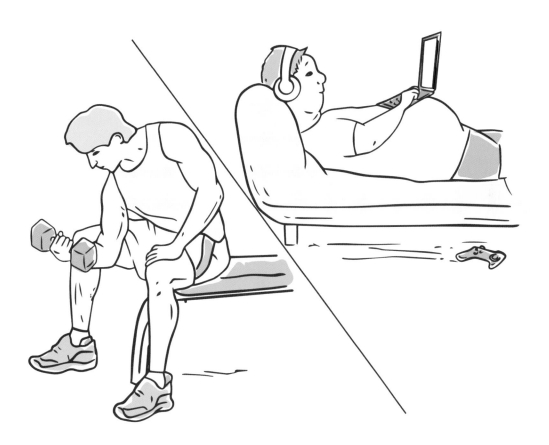

Ted, an active person who weighs 175 pounds, goes to the gym four or five days a week, has a decent amount of muscle mass, has a fasting blood sugar level of 87—that's healthy—and has no signs of inflammation. He wants to try keto because he wants to turn his body into a metabolic machine that easily taps into his fat stores for fuel. He wants to be able to go longer without eating, stop getting hangry, and see how his brain feels on keto.

Then we have Austin, who is not active and weighs 295 pounds. He doesn't lift weights, has a fasting blood sugar level of 120 (considered prediabetic on the verge of diabetic), has a lot of aches and pains in his joints, feels mentally foggy, and borders on depressed. He wants to do keto to lose weight and feel good again.

These two will have very different experiences on a ketogenic diet. Because Ted already has good blood sugar management, he will likely feel *somewhat* weak as his body transitions into ketosis. However, since the effect will be barely felt, Ted likely won't find the transition to be that difficult. Austin, on the other hand, will probably feel like garbage in the beginning. Those first few days on keto are likely going to be hard for him. His body is not used to running on its own fat practically *ever;* it is entirely dependent on glucose for energy. So, when Austin stops giving his body a nonstop supply of glucose, it's going to freak out a little. He will be much more likely than Ted to experience the "keto flu" (weakness, lethargy, and feeling almost sick), although Ted might experience it, too, if he normally eats a lot of carbs and eats frequently.

After the first few days, they both should start to feel more normal and experience more balanced energy throughout the day. Without blood sugar highs and lows, afternoon dips in energy will begin to dissipate. As their bodies realize they can just run on their own fat for fuel, both Ted and Austin will feel like they can go much longer between meals without feeling hungry. As their brains start receiving ketones as an energy source, they may feel a new sense of mental clarity, especially if they had some brain glucose metabolism issues they weren't aware of. (As we age, we lose the ability to metabolize glucose as effectively in our brains, which leads to feelings of brain fog, decreased memory, and less focus. However, we never lose the ability to use ketones as a brain energy source. This brings more mental clarity to those who may have some impaired brain glucose metabolism—likely without realizing it—when they go on a ketogenic diet.)

Austin will likely start to notice that his chronic pain is going away, his weight is dropping steadily, his energy levels are up, and his fasted blood sugar is going down. He will probably become a huge fan of the ketogenic diet because he's going to feel and look better than he ever has.

Ted might notice less achiness in his joints; he may drop a little bit of body fat and enjoy a little more mental clarity. However, keto is unlikely to be a life-changing experience for him since he already has good blood sugar management. Ted might also notice a decrease in athletic performance and have a slightly more difficult time building muscle. All this might be a cool experiment for Ted, but he likely won't become a keto enthusiast the way Austin will. After all, Ted feels just about the same on keto as he does when he eats healthy carbohydrates, which is also when he gets to train more intensely and grow muscle a little more easily.

In short, much of the keto experience depends on a person's metabolic environment when they start. People who are already metabolically healthy probably won't have the mind-blowing experience on keto that people with metabolic dysfunction experience.

This brings us to the point of this chapter: do we need to do keto forever when our metabolisms are healthy?

Let's dig in. In this chapter, I cover the following topics:

- Why not stay keto forever?
- What can go wrong if you stay keto too long
- How long you should do keto
- The benefits of eating carbohydrates and why you might consider increasing them after a keto phase
- Restoring your relationship with carbs after keto
- Biofeedback to look for when increasing carbohydrates

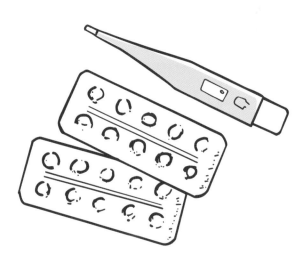

WHY NOT STAY
KETO FOREVER?

Before I begin discussing why I don't think staying keto forever is optimal for most people, I'd like to explain what happens inside your body after you eat carbohydrates and after you eat fat so you have a foundational understanding. It's amazing how much easier it is to make intelligent food choices when you know what foods actually do once they get inside your body! We tend to fear things we don't understand, and most people seem to have *no idea* how carbohydrates work in their own bodies. All they know is that they've heard a lot of bad things about carbs lately—specifically, the message that carbs will make you fat.

So let's dig in. Do they? Do carbs "make you fat"?

Let's cover a little science so you understand what happens in your body after you eat carbohydrates. Here's how it goes in a nutshell:

You eat carbs. Your blood sugar goes up. Let's call it "blood energy" instead of "blood sugar" for this example. The term "blood sugar" has gotten a terrible reputation, so I don't want to call it that. What is the "sugar" in your blood? It's energy! It's the little molecules of energy that fuel every single cell in your entire body (as long as you aren't insulin resistant, which I will discuss momentarily). That energy is going to be shuttled all over your body to power your cells: your brain, heart, organs, muscles—everything. What your body can't use immediately for fuel, it stores. But where does it store it?

These days, everyone seems to think excess energy is immediately stored as body fat. But that's far from the truth. Your body stores extra carbohydrates as glycogen in your liver and muscles first and *then* stores any extra as body fat.

This is absolutely key to understand: your body stores a lot of carbohydrates in other places before it goes to body fat! There is an important middleman here—a holding tank, a buffer—and it's crucial to know this about your body.

Your liver can hold about 100 to 120 grams of glycogen. Your muscles can hold even more. The average person stores roughly 350 to 500 grams of glycogen in their muscles. The exact amount your body can store depends on how much muscle mass you have, of course. Trained athletes can store up to 700 grams of glycogen in their muscles.[2] This is one of the reasons people with more muscle mass seem to "get away with murder" in regard to how many carbs they can eat and not get fat. They just have bigger storage tanks! Besides, they are engaging in weight training, and most likely cardiovascular exercise as well, both of which empty those storage tanks often, making room for more carbs.

It's only when the storage space for glycogen in the muscles and liver is full that the liver converts the extra carbohydrates to body fat. That is quite the buffer between consumption of carbohydrates and body fat storage. (You don't get that with dietary fat, by the way, as I will discuss shortly.)

But first, let me be abundantly clear: unless you are insulin resistant, it's not carbohydrates that make you fat; it is an excess of carbohydrates. And you get a lot of leeway before that happens. On top of the "middleman" (your liver and muscles), your brain consumes about 20 percent of the carbohydrates you eat before the excess gets stored as body fat. After that, if you don't go long enough between meals to use up the excess, or if you don't exercise enough to use up the excess, you just keep that body fat. And this happens over and over again with every overeating session until you gradually become overweight or obese.

Okay, now, let's talk about what happens when you eat fat. Dietary fat is much more easily stored as body fat than carbohydrates. Very little dietary fat is stored in the muscles and liver. You don't get a giant buffer between consumption and fat storage! We don't know exactly how much fat is stored in the muscles and liver, but it is a much smaller amount. And the more fat you store in your liver and muscles, the more predisposed you are to developing a fatty liver, becoming obese, developing type 2 diabetes, and creating disease states.

Therefore, even though they can do so to a minimal extent, our bodies try not to store much fat in the muscles and liver; instead, they send the bulk of excess dietary fat straight to the fat cells in our adipose tissue, or what we commonly refer to as "body fat," both visceral (the dangerous fat around our organs) and subcutaneous (the body fat that makes us look fat).

> Dietary fat is also stored much more efficiently; storing carbs as fat burns a lot more calories than storing dietary fat as fat. Let's say you eat 100 calories' (25 grams') worth of excess carbohydrates. It takes 23 calories' worth of energy to convert that glucose to fat and then store it as body fat. But if you eat 100 calories' (about 11 grams') worth of excess dietary fat, it takes only 2.5 calories to store it as body fat. As you can see, dietary fat is stored as body fat ten times more efficiently than carbohydrates.[3]

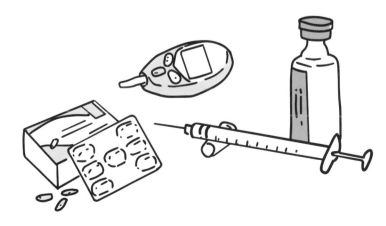

So remember, when you eat fat, you don't get a buffer between eating and fat storage like you do when you eat carbohydrates. Almost all of the dietary fat you eat that isn't immediately used for energy is stored as body fat.

The only caveat is when you are in a ketogenic state. Being in a ketogenic state flips a metabolic switch that causes your body to prioritize dietary fat as its energy source. That basically means that without carbohydrates, you will need more fat to operate your body, so you can eat more fat than usual without gaining body fat. In a ketogenic state, your liver glycogen is low because you're eating barely any carbs. Knowing it has to get energy from somewhere, your body starts processing dietary fat quickly into ketones for energy. However, when you're not in ketosis and there is enough liver glycogen for your body to use as fuel, you won't need as much fat. Any excess is then quickly and easily stored as body fat.

This is so important to understand. I see many people gain quite a bit of body fat after doing keto because they're still eating a lot of fat even after bringing carbs back in. I also see people gain body fat from doing "lazy keto," meaning they are "sort of eating keto" without consciously restricting carbohydrates enough to ensure that they're in a ketogenic state. What often happens is that they consume a lot of fat without actually being in ketosis. Their bodies are trying to run on glycogen because they are eating just enough carbs to prevent ketosis, but since there's very little glycogen available, they experience low energy levels. This is not a good place to be. Also, because they're eating tons of fat without having flipped the metabolic switch to favor fat as the primary energy source, that dietary fat just goes to fat storage. It's a common problem, and it leads to a lot of frustration and fat-loss plateaus. And if a person isn't restricting calories, it can easily lead to fat gain while "eating keto." I experienced this myself when I first went keto, and I've seen it time and time again in others. Word to the wise.

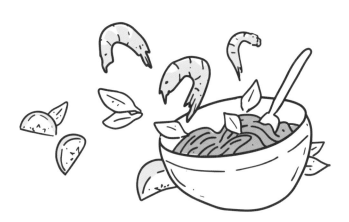

WHAT ABOUT INSULIN RESISTANCE?

Now, I told you I would discuss insulin resistance. This is another important piece of this puzzle to understand, because it changes things.

What is insulin resistance? I like to use an analogy here because I think it makes this subject easier to understand.

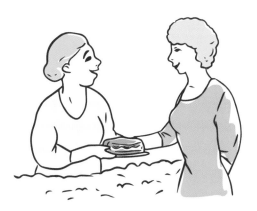

Imagine that you've just moved into a new house. Everything is amazing, except you haven't gone grocery shopping yet and don't have any food. You're getting pretty hungry, but you're also very busy unpacking and organizing.

Like a godsend, your next-door neighbor shows up at the perfect time with a big slice of chocolate cake to welcome you to the neighborhood. Your neighbor in this example is insulin, the cake is glucose, and your house is one of your cells.

You gratefully accept the cake and eat it. It gives you tons of energy to continue unpacking and organizing.

A couple of hours later, your neighbor shows up with two more slices of cake. You find it kind of surprising (and maybe a little weird). You are admittedly hungry again, though, so you accept those slices of cake with gratitude and proceed to eat both of them.

An hour later, this same neighbor shows up with five slices of cake. You know there is no way you can eat five more slices. You awkwardly accept one piece but tell her you can't possibly eat five slices and send her away with the other four. You suggest that she offer them to the other neighbors. You eat that slice of cake and find yourself absolutely stuffed.

An hour later, she shows up again with eight slices of cake. What in the world...? You realize you're going to have to set some boundaries, so you tell her no, thanks—you don't want any cake. And you send her away.

Before long, you realize this is going to become a regular thing: she brings you cake all day, every day—sometimes even at midnight. Many months pass, and the cake deliveries continue. And because the cake is really good, you still accept it sometimes. But you're definitely building up some resistance to this annoying neighbor and her constant onslaught of dessert. Most of the time, you just don't answer the door.

However, because your neighbor believes you really need cake, she gets worried and enlists the help of her family. Soon, you have even more cake deliveries coming to your door, and you just can't take it anymore. You've built up a heavy resistance to this cake delivery. You stop answering the door entirely.

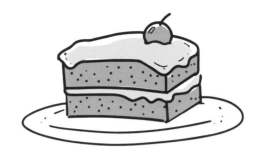

I share this somewhat silly example to illustrate how our cells become resistant to something that they once considered really great. Our cells, which once loved glucose and gladly answered the door when insulin came knocking, have just had way too much. So, as they start to see the delivery guy as a threat, they build up a resistance to insulin.

Then system-wide miscommunication begins. Now that our cells aren't taking in as much glucose, our blood sugar levels go up. That's a big problem, and it can have a bunch of drastic consequences in the body—including, you know, stuff like death. So our pancreas says: *I must need to make more insulin!*

The pancreas sends out more and more insulin—more delivery guys—and the insulin can't find enough cells to take all this glucose. As a result, the body creates new cells—fat cells—to have somewhere to put it all.

As this cycle continues for years, the body becomes confused, thinking it needs more carbs because cellular energy is low. So, desperate for energy, it demands lots of carbs and produces tons of insulin because that's what it has learned to do. And when the glucose can't get into the muscle and organ cells because they have become insulin resistant, the insulin has nowhere to put the glucose except in fat cells. And so this person lives a life of low energy, high hunger, and high fat storage. This is how obesity, type 2 diabetes, and metabolic dysfunction happen.

All of this opens up an interesting discussion about whether or not carbs are a useful part of a fat-loss diet. If you are insulin resistant, carbs are not going to be your friend for fat loss or for energy levels. Instead of fueling your muscle and organ cells, a large amount of the carbs you eat will go to your fat cells.

A ketogenic diet is, for this reason, a highly effective dietary intervention for anyone who has insulin resistance. The ketone bodies will fuel the cells, so the insulin-resistant person will finally have energy again. They'll almost certainly lose body fat because there aren't excess carbs to be put away in their fat stores anymore. Not only that, but the fat they eat will be favored for ketone production instead of going to storage like it would when eating a carb-heavy diet. Insulin resistance improves quickly for most people once they begin a ketogenic diet, and the reason for that appears to be the actual ketone bodies, not just the reduction in carbohydrates.[4]

This is why we see so many obese people raving about the results they got from keto. It is the only thing that has worked for them. The Uber driver who drove me to KetoCon in Austin, Texas, in 2019, was one of them. When she found out where I was headed, she proceeded to tell me that she had lost 150 pounds on keto. Prior to that, she had been morbidly obese; she was housebound and had given up on life. Keto was the only thing that ever worked for her, and she was so grateful for it. And now, on top of her Uber job, she had started her own catering company and had a new lease on life.

These are the kinds of stories I hear over and over from obese people who have done keto. My obese clients love how keto gets their blood sugar regulated straight out of the gate so they're not having highs and lows and restores insulin sensitivity so they stop storing so much body fat. They've found this way of eating to be life-changing!

But what do you do when you have become insulin sensitive again and are metabolically healthy? This is what I really want to get across in this book. Once you've restored insulin sensitivity, the game changes! You don't have to pigeonhole yourself into keto forever when doing so is likely to be unnecessary. Recognize that you are no longer in the same body! Your metabolism has changed! You did some deep, amazing work on your metabolism. Good for you! But what you needed when you were insulin resistant is likely not needed anymore when you are insulin sensitive.

This concept is really tough for people to accept mentally and emotionally. I understand that if you lose 100 pounds by not eating carbohydrates, you're going to be pretty dead set on never eating them again. I totally get it! But don't get caught in that trap.

Find out what your fasting glucose and hemoglobin A1c (HbA1c) are. If they're within the normal ranges, you can slowly start reintroducing carbohydrates. Please make them whole-food carbohydrates from nature! Fiber is important. Fiber also helps increase insulin sensitivity. It helps us remain insulin sensitive long term and offers a host of health benefits. If you reintroduce carbs by eating every junk-food

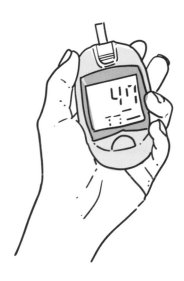

carb that exists because you've been restricting so long that you totally go off the rails, well, you're going to feel horrible. Those carbs are not the carbs I'm talking about. I'm talking about unprocessed carbs from nature, like vegetables, fruits, and whole grains. They're totally different things.

Now, how long does this process take? How do you even know if you're insulin resistant? And how do you know when you've become insulin sensitive again? Two blood tests will give you the answer:

- A fasting glucose test tells you what your blood sugar level is on that day.

- An HbA1c test tells you what your blood sugar regulation has looked like over the past few months.

What are the healthy ranges? According to the American Diabetes Association, a fasting blood glucose level under 100 mg/dL is considered normal. However, a 2008 study found that people with a fasting blood glucose level of 95 to 99 were 2.33 times more likely to develop diabetes.[5] Another study of metabolically healthy people showed that they had, on average, a fasting blood glucose of 89.3 mg/dL.[6] I recommend getting your fasting glucose level under 90 mg/dL before reincorporating carbohydrates.

A healthy HbA1c is under 5.7 percent, but studies have shown that under 5.0 percent is ideal for preventing heart disease, and one study found that anything over 4.6 percent was associated with an increased risk of heart disease.[7] Anything between 5.7 and 6.5 percent is considered prediabetic by the American Diabetes Association, and anything above that is considered diabetic.

How long the insulin resistance lasts is very individual, and factors such as the duration of the insulin resistance and physical activity level may play a part in how well a person will be able to tolerate carbohydrates after they are reintroduced. While most people don't need to stay keto forever, people with persistent insulin resistance may find it an optimal lifestyle choice.

How do you know if you have insulin resistance? Have your fasting blood glucose and HbA1c checked. Elevated levels of these biomarkers are indicative of insulin resistance. Once they are within normal ranges, it is likely that you have restored insulin sensitivity.

Keto is an incredibly powerful tool for restoring insulin sensitivity. I've had clients with a fasting blood sugar level of over 100 mg/dL drop into the eighties in less than a year, even after the reintroduction of more carbs following a phase of keto. It works. Lowering your carb intake alone can help resensitize you to insulin, but doing a ketogenic diet is going to be even better, as you'll have a new energy source from ketone bodies that your cells can actually use.

As a quick aside, please be aware that for a couple of weeks after reintroducing carbohydrates, your insulin sensitivity might appear to be low. This effect is temporary. Your blood sugar may shoot up after you eat a meal containing carbs, probably because your body is not used to producing enough insulin to handle a normal level of carbohydrate consumption. However, your system will normalize within two weeks.

A study published in the journal *Endocrinology* compared rats that ate "normal chow" (a combination of protein, fat, and carbohydrates) with rats that ate a ketogenic diet for eight weeks. After eight weeks, both groups were fed high-carbohydrate meals. The ketogenic rats had elevated insulin levels when tested 120 minutes after the meal, while the normal-chow rats did not. For the ketogenic rats, glucose increased within fifteen minutes of the high-carbohydrate meal and remained elevated and unchanged from its peak level at the 120-minute point. Their ability to respond appropriately to a high-carbohydrate meal was impaired. This lasted for only one week, and then the insulin and glucose response in the rats that had been ketogenic was restored to normal, to the same rate as the rats that had always been fed standard chow.[8]

So, once insulin sensitivity has been re-established and is verified by healthy fasting blood glucose and HbA1c levels, it's a good time to gradually increase healthy carbohydrates in your diet and see how your body responds. As you will see in the meal plan in Appendix C, you gradually increase carbohydrates over a period of four weeks to give your digestive system time to gently adjust to the change in macronutrients. At the end of the four weeks, you will be getting only 25 percent of your calories from fat and 35 percent of your calories from carbs. This amount of carbohydrates can make keto dieters fearful that they will gain body fat. So, although they're often willing to eat "a little more carbs," they still want to stay high fat and low carb. But is eating a high-fat, low-carb (but not keto) diet a wise approach for achieving fat loss and/or preventing fat gain, especially when you are insulin sensitive?

I say no, it's not. Here's why:

If you can eat carbs and shuttle them into your cells normally, with somewhere around 500 grams of carbs (that's 2,000 calories) being stored in your liver and muscles, plus 20 percent of your carbs being used by your brain for energy, all before any carbs go to fat storage, doesn't that sound like carbohydrates might be an intelligent macronutrient choice in terms of preventing body fat storage?

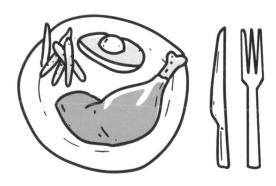

Dietary fat, on the other hand, doesn't have the enormous "middleman" between consumption and fat storage that carbs do. When you eat fat, you use it immediately, and any extra is stored as body fat.

On top of this, carbohydrates are the primary fuel for intense exercise and help build muscle. Fat is not a building block of muscle. Sure, it helps indirectly by boosting testosterone production, but how much fat do we really need? What is the bare minimum amount of fat needed for optimal human health? What's our baseline here?

First, understand that fat is essential. You will die if you never eat it. That would be pretty hard to do, though, considering that even plants such as raspberries and rice contain small amounts of fat.

The dietary reference intake (DRI) for adults is 20 to 35 percent of total calories from fat. That is about 44 to 77 grams of fat per day if you eat 2,000 calories a day, or 33 to 58 grams if you eat 1,500 calories a day.[9] It's impossible to give an exact number of daily fat grams needed for all humans since we all have different genetics, age, activity level, hormonal environments, and other health factors, but this gives us a ballpark.

We need to take in enough fat for vital body functions, such as absorbing fat-soluble vitamins, building healthy cells, maintaining healthy brain and nervous system function, proper immune function, reproductive health, energy production, hormone health, and healthy cholesterol production. The question is: once we have consumed enough fat for our bodies to do those things properly, do we really need to be eating much more, especially when we are trying to lose body fat or prevent extra fat storage? Also, how much fat do we really need beyond what's necessary when we are not in a ketogenic state where our bodies are using the fat as their primary energy source?

This issue needs to be discussed because it seems these days that anything marketed as "low carb" is deemed a health food, much like low-fat foods were marketed as health foods in the 1990s.

Just like in the 1990s, when food companies compensated for the low fat content in their products with excess sugar, most low-carb food companies today are compensating with excess fat. I want you to be mindful of what was discussed earlier, which is that if you're not actually on a ketogenic diet, when you eat more fat than your body needs at any given moment, most of that excess goes straight to fat storage!

Let's compare apples to apples with these "healthy" ice creams: one marketed as high protein and the other marketed as keto. The Halo Top brand is a higher-protein, lower-calorie ice cream, but it's too high in carbs to be considered a low-carb product. The Rebel brand is very low in net carbs but very high in fat.

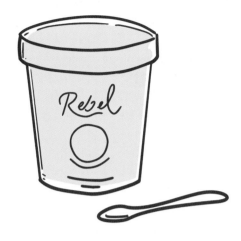

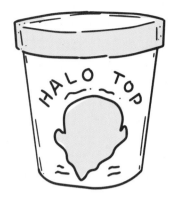

1 PINT OF VANILLA REBEL KETO ICE CREAM

Calories: 560

Fat: 56g

Saturated fat: 34g

Protein: 6g

Carbohydrates: 38g

Fiber (subtract from carbs): 7g

Erythritol (subtract from carbs): 27g

Net carbs: 4g

1 PINT OF VANILLA HALO TOP PROTEIN ICE CREAM

Calories: 290

Fat: 6g

Saturated fat: 3.5g

Protein: 19g

Carbohydrates: 62g

Fiber (subtract from carbs): 17g

Erythritol (subtract from carbs): 23g

Net carbs: 22g

As you can see, the Halo Top brand has

- Nearly half the calories
- More than three times the protein
- More than double the fiber
- More than five times the net carbs

So, assuming you are not insulin resistant, when it comes to fat loss, which ice cream is more likely to give you both an immediate and a prolonged sense of fullness for fewer calories? According to research on satiety, the Halo Top will, even though it has more than five times the net carbs. Why?

First of all, protein and carbohydrates have the biggest impact on suppressing ghrelin, the hunger hormone. A 2010 study examining the impact each of the macronutrients has on suppressing ghrelin found that carbohydrates were the most effective for immediate ghrelin suppression, protein was the most effective for prolonged ghrelin suppression (and the most satiating of the three macronutrients), and fat exhibited a weak and insufficient ghrelin-suppressing capacity.[10]

Secondly, the Rebel ice cream is high in animal-based saturated fat (from cream). In a study published in the *Journal of Clinical Investigation,* the researchers found that after only three days on a diet high in saturated fat—a common component of animal fats—the brains of rats and mice became resistant to leptin (our satiety hormone) and insulin.[11] If the same thing happens in humans, regularly eating meals high in saturated fat could potentially crank up appetite.

Another study looked into the impact of high-protein and high-fat snacks on satiety. It found high-protein snacks to be more effective for improving appetite control and satiety and reducing food intake in the next meal.[12]

And don't forget that the high-protein Halo Top ice cream has nearly half the calories! So you're more satiated on fewer calories. This combination of high protein and low calories is crucial for fat loss, and it is something every person who wants to lose body fat should be mindful of.

Now that we have established that carbs are not the enemy of fat loss, let's dive into the other reasons I don't recommend doing keto for the rest of your life.

Here are a few of them:

- Increased risk of nutritional deficiencies
- Chronically elevated adrenaline
- Hair loss
- Decreased ability to build muscle
- Likelihood of putting on body fat because you're not actually in ketosis but still eating large amounts of fat
- Decreased microbial diversity in the gut
- Hindered exercise performance
- Chronic risk of electrolyte/mineral imbalance
- Potentially low serotonin levels
- Possible negative effects on sleep
- Binge eating/disordered eating patterns

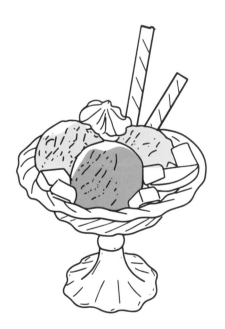

Going through a phase of keto, namely intermittent bouts of metabolizing body fat into ketone bodies, is great for your metabolism. But doing keto all the time, forever? Now you've swung the metabolic pendulum toward the other extreme, once again pigeonholing your metabolism into a fraction of its potential.

The goal is metabolic flexibility. You want a metabolism that can easily transition between glycolysis and ketosis, rather than a metabolism that is limited to one or the other. That means you can eat carbohydrates and operate optimally or go without them and also operate optimally.

Ask yourself these questions: If you don't need your glycolytic system, why do you have it? More significantly, if you don't need your glycolytic system, why does your body use that one first, going into ketosis only in the absence (or extreme limitation) of carbohydrates?

Human bodies like carbohydrates. Actually, let me be more specific: *when you're healthy,* your body loves carbohydrates. In a normal, healthy human metabolism, the body thrives on healthy carbohydrates.

The problem is, if you are sick and inflamed from years of processed foods, toxins, stress, and sleep deprivation, your body no longer metabolizes carbohydrates effectively. If your gut is inflamed, your cells are insulin resistant, and your blood sugar is already high, carbs are not going to be your friend, and your body is not going to love carbs. This is why I advocate for a phase of keto for many people. It's extremely healing. It can restore insulin sensitivity, resolve a lot of gut issues, get blood sugar levels back to normal, reduce inflammation, and prepare the body to be a healthy metabolizer of carbohydrates once again.

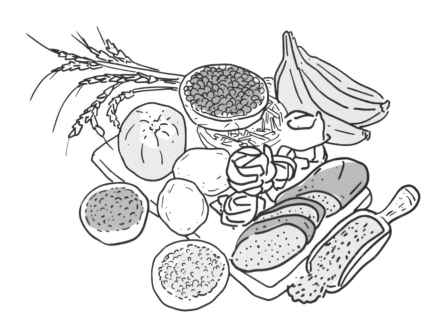

Many keto advocates who tell you that carbs don't love you back are people coming at this subject from the therapeutic angle. Many of these people used keto to heal, and many have ongoing health issues that are not triggered when they are in ketosis, so of course they become evangelists for the diet. If keto healed your autoimmunity or your cancer, you're going to be a pretty big fan!

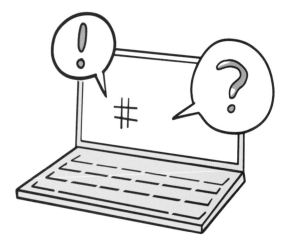

While I wholeheartedly support ketogenic dieting as a therapeutic tool for a variety of illnesses, my question is this: What about the people who don't have any of these conditions but just want to optimize their metabolisms, lose some weight, and feel great?

The messages these people receive when they go online for help are

- Carbs will make you fat.
- Carbs will inflame you.
- Carbs are trying to kill you. (Yes, even that one.)

So people go on their keto diet adventure. For some, it's life-changing! Many of these people had issues like insulin resistance or high inflammation and didn't even know it.

But for many, the adventure doesn't lead them to a great place. Not even close. Allow me to be the whistleblower from inside the keto community when I say that keto does not work for everyone. For some, it is a nightmare. These people gain weight, feel worse, can't sleep, don't recover fully from their workouts, and have terrible digestion—the list goes on.

I have worked one-on-one with hundreds of people. Some absolutely thrive on keto, and others definitely do better when they eat more carbs. And when my keto clients reintroduce healthy carbs at the right time, they continue to lose weight, feel great, and usually comment on how much better their workouts are. I generally notice more calmness in their demeanor now that their blood sugar has been regulated, which I will go into in just a moment.

Dr. Mark Hyman, an internationally recognized authority in the low-carb community and the author of the books *Eat Fat, Get Thin* and *The Blood Sugar Solution*, has said this:

"I have something surprising to say that might go against everything you've heard: Carbs are the single most important thing you can eat for health and weight loss. In fact, I often say my plan is a high-carb diet.

But wait, you say, don't carbs contribute to insulin resistance, heart disease, and other health concerns?

Some do, but the truth is more complicated. You see, "carbohydrates" encompasses a huge category. A hot fudge sundae and cauliflower both fall into the "carbs" category, yet they are entirely different foods.

In fact, almost all plant foods fall into the carbs category. These are what I refer to as slow carbs, which are low-glycemic and don't spike your blood sugar or insulin. These slow carbs come loaded with nutrients, fiber, and amazing molecules called phytochemicals.

When you eat a cornucopia of fresh fruits and vegetables teeming with phytonutrients—carotenoids, flavonoids, and polyphenols—they help improve nearly all health problems, including dementia, diabesity, and aging.

Ideally, about 75% of your carb intake should come from nonstarchy veggies plus low-glycemic fruits. By volume, most of your plate should be carbs. Note I said volume, not calories. Many plant-based carbs actually have very few calories."[13]

Dr. Hyman brings up a great point, and I wholeheartedly agree with him. I cannot emphasize enough that

- We cannot lump all carbs together.
- We cannot suggest that Twinkies fall into the same category as potatoes.
- Real, unprocessed carbohydrates from nature impact the body in an entirely different way than candy bars.

Before I get into how carbohydrates can help you lose weight, perform better in the gym, and feel better overall, let's look at some reasons keto might actually hold you back from getting the body composition results you're after.

WHAT CAN GO WRONG
IF YOU STAY ON
KETO TOO LONG

There are some possible drawbacks to staying on a ketogenic diet long term that you should be aware of. It's common for me to see people feel really amazing on keto at first while some things get corrected in their body. However, as time goes on, they progressively begin to feel less good than they once did. In this section, I will discuss some of those potential concerns.

CHANGES IN YOUR NEUROCHEMISTRY MAY HAVE SERIOUS PSYCHOLOGICAL CONSEQUENCES

If there is one thing I want to shout from the rooftops in this book, it's this: Your food choices alter your neurochemistry.

And because we all have different baseline neurotransmitter levels (meaning I might be naturally high in something that you are naturally low in), drastically altering the macronutrients we eat can have a significant impact on our mental and emotional well-being. Extreme changes to your macronutrient ratios will have an effect on your mental state. This is incredibly important to know!

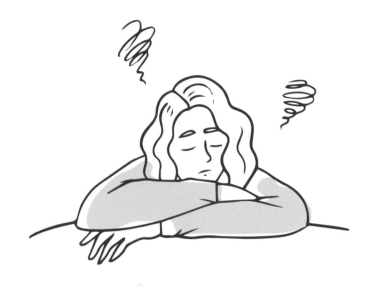

Keto's impact on dopamine and serotonin is something I would like people to understand at a broader level. These are the two neurotransmitters most often associated with mental health issues and mood. When you're on a ketogenic diet, your body makes more dopamine and less serotonin. When it comes to people for whom this shift works out well, keto is great. However, for people who need more serotonin but don't need more dopamine, keto can be a very negative experience.

Too often, I've seen people be overly hard on themselves because they don't feel mentally well on keto and keep "caving" to carb cravings. These people often believe that there's something wrong with them—that they just don't have enough willpower. Let's address that point right this second (said in my best sternly loving mom voice).

Our neurotransmitters heavily affect our mood and our choices; they basically create our personalities. Not to wound your ego, but you're unlikely to win a battle of willpower against your neurochemistry. Let's start with a foundational understanding.

First, what are neurotransmitters? They are the chemicals in our brains that impact how we show up in life. When people talk about chemical imbalances, they are referring to neurotransmitters. Our neurotransmitters are the chemical messengers that tell our bodies what to do.

There are over 100 different neurotransmitters, but these seven main neurotransmitters do the majority of the work:

- Acetylcholine
- Adrenaline (epinephrine)
- Dopamine
- Gamma-aminobutyric acid (GABA)
- Glutamate
- Oxytocin
- Serotonin

Eating a ketogenic diet significantly impacts the levels of five of these important neurotransmitters: glutamate, GABA, dopamine, serotonin, and adrenaline.

Let's discuss what each one does and how they are affected by a ketogenic diet versus a carbohydrate-rich diet.

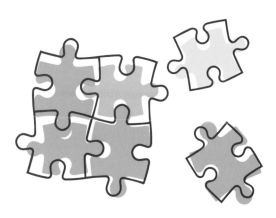

GLUTAMATE

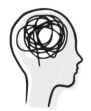

Glutamate is a common amino acid in food. It acts as an excitatory neurotransmitter; that is to say, it stimulates neurons to fire commands. It's present in 90 percent of synapses (the small space between neurons, or brain/nervous system cells, where they communicate with each other). Glutamate is important. However, when we have too much of it, our neurons get overstimulated. This results in feelings of anxiety and uncontrollable, racing thoughts. Some people have an underactive glutamic acid decarboxylase (GAD) enzyme, the enzyme that helps us convert glutamate to GABA, our main inhibitory neurotransmitter, which stops racing thoughts and helps us relax and feel cool, calm, and collected.

A person who has high amounts of glutamate may experience the following:

- Anxiety
- Muscle pain
- Addiction
- A tendency to be overly hard on themselves
- Mood swings
- Overthinking/racing thoughts
- Difficulty concentrating
- Insomnia

Studies have found that ketogenic diets help increase the conversion of glutamate to GABA.[14] So, if someone is experiencing anxiety or racing thoughts because of an excess of glutamate, they may feel better mentally when they switch to keto.

GABA

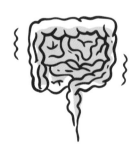

GABA is glutamate's polar opposite. It is the main inhibitory neurotransmitter of the nervous system, reducing activity of the central nervous system like the brake pedal for our brain.

Scientists estimate that nearly all GABA is manufactured in the gut, thereby establishing a connection between the gut and the brain. Poor gut health, therefore, makes it difficult for your body to make the proper amount of GABA. And if you don't have enough GABA, you will feel stressed and anxious, which can lower the levels of GABA in your gut even more. So managing stress, eating a healthy diet, and exercising are all correlated with higher GABA levels. What's interesting is that you have to eat foods that are high in glutamate in order to have healthy GABA levels, but if your conversion from glutamate to GABA is poor, you'll just be anxious and stressed from eating these foods.

Making sure you have adequate levels of vitamin B6 is important, as it is a co-factor in converting glutamate to GABA. Fermented foods also feed the healthy bacteria in your gut that synthesize GABA, so foods that are rich in probiotics, like sauerkraut, kimchi, miso, yogurt, and kefir, can help raise GABA levels as well. The probiotics *Lactobacillus rhamnosus, Lactobacillus paracasei, Lactobacillus brevis,* and *Lactococcus lactis* have been shown to boost the production of GABA.[15]

Symptoms of low GABA include anxiety, depression, insomnia, and mood disorders. The more GABA you have, the more self-control you have and the more relaxed you feel. For these reasons, people with low GABA levels tend to feel much better mentally on keto. But those who already have high GABA levels won't experience these benefits.

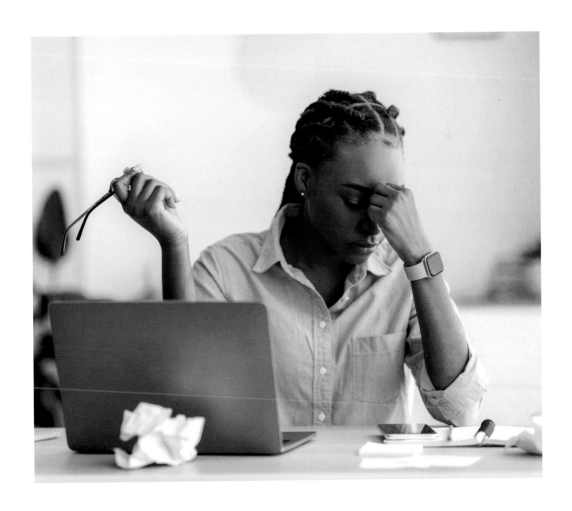

DOPAMINE

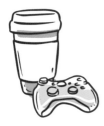

Dopamine helps us feel happy, confident, driven, and outgoing; it just helps us feel that good feeling—pleasure. It's considered the reward chemical. Many drugs and common mood enhancers, such as caffeine, raise dopamine levels. Even addictive activities like gaming, gambling, shopping, and working out can create dopamine highs.

Low dopamine levels, on the other hand, can lead to feelings of depression and apathy. People with low dopamine may have low mood, low sex drive, fatigue, attention difficulties, chronic pain, weight fluctuations, and even mental health issues such as major depressive disorder, schizophrenia, and the neurological disease Parkinson's disease. Type 2 diabetes can also cause low dopamine.

Ketogenic diets have been shown to raise dopamine levels, which can be very beneficial for people with low dopamine.[16] However, those who already have higher baseline dopamine levels may experience extremely high libido, anxiety, difficulty sleeping, mania, and stress when dopamine is further increased. High baseline dopamine levels are often evident in personality traits like confidence, quick decision making, extroversion, energy, enthusiasm, and mental flexibility, so be aware that if you already have high dopamine, a ketogenic diet can potentially send you into an über-confident, high-anxiety, stressed state.

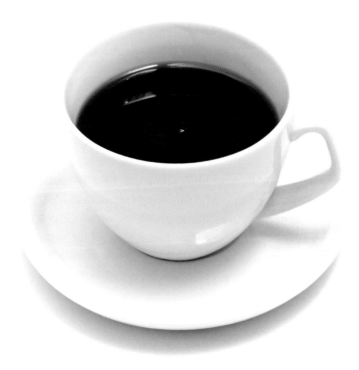

SEROTONIN

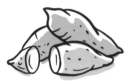

Low carbohydrate consumption over long periods of time can result in low serotonin levels. For people who are already predisposed to low serotonin, this further drop on keto can result in a series of mental health issues, including disordered eating patterns or eating disorders, anxiety, depressed mood, aggression, impulsive behavior, insomnia, irritability, crying spells, low self-esteem, and poor appetite.

The emotion that is heightened with low serotonin is guilt, which can contribute even more to disordered eating patterns on a ketogenic diet. So, if you are experiencing these symptoms on keto, it may be wise to switch to a diet with more carbohydrates. Carbohydrates help the amino acid tryptophan enter the brain, where it is converted to serotonin. Very little tryptophan is able to cross the blood-brain barrier unless carbohydrate is present. Carbohydrate consumption causes the body to release more insulin, which promotes amino acid absorption and leaves tryptophan in the blood. If protein is consumed with carbohydrates, the carbohydrates will help drive the tryptophan in the protein across the blood-brain barrier much more easily. So, while people who have good baseline levels of serotonin may feel good mentally on keto, people who have low baseline levels can experience negative psychological effects on a ketogenic diet.

ADRENALINE (EPINEPHRINE)

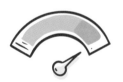

Because the body excretes sodium at a much faster rate on a ketogenic diet, and people are often unsure if they are replenishing sodium adequately, they run the risk of having increased adrenaline levels on keto, which happens when we don't have sufficient circulating sodium in our blood. Active people who sweat a lot on a ketogenic diet, who live in areas with hot weather, and who drink a lot of caffeine, which also depletes sodium, are even more at risk for high adrenaline on keto. This can lead to anxiety and poor sleep, not to mention high cortisol levels.

So, while high adrenaline can be offset with proper sodium balance, people who are living high-stress lifestyles, don't know their sodium levels, and are following a ketogenic diet can run into problems. They may love the feeling of high energy, but being high on adrenaline all the time can have negative health consequences. If you are feeling anxious and jittery and have poor sleep on keto, it may be wise to bring back the carbs.

In summary, pay attention to how your diet is affecting your mood. So often, we forget that the two are related.

YOU MAY DEVELOP ADRENAL ISSUES, ELECTROLYTE IMBALANCES, AND HIGH CORTISOL

Stephen Phinney and Jeff Volek, two of the leading researchers on the ketogenic diet, have found that people who don't carefully monitor sodium and potassium while on keto can run into adrenal issues.[17] Here's how it happens:

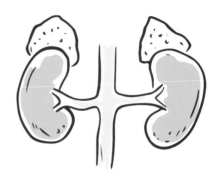

When you're in a ketogenic state, your kidneys switch from retaining sodium to rapidly excreting it,[18] making sodium deficiency likely if you're not monitoring it carefully. Sodium deficiency is a big deal. If you don't get any sodium for more than a few weeks, you'll die.

Aside from death as the most serious outcome, what other things can happen if you become sodium deficient? Your adrenal glands make a hormone called aldosterone that causes your kidneys to conserve sodium but simultaneously waste potassium. So that leads you to become potassium deficient.

Potassium deficiency can be dangerous as well. Without sufficient potassium, your muscles, heart, and nerves cannot work properly. If you're experiencing muscle spasms and heart palpitations on keto, there's a good chance that you could be potassium deficient. Ask your doctor to check your sodium and potassium levels.

On top of the risk of potassium deficiency, low sodium increases adrenal production of the stress hormone cortisol and the fight-or-flight hormone adrenaline. What happens when you have chronically elevated cortisol and adrenaline? Elevated cortisol results in

- Increased blood sugar levels
- Weight gain
- Suppression of body functions that aren't essential in a fight-or-flight situation
- Suppression of your immune system
- Digestive problems
- Low libido, erectile dysfunction, irregular ovulation or menstrual cycle
- Difficulty recovering from exercise
- Poor sleep

Cortisol also communicates with the regions of the brain that control mood, motivation, and fear, so chronically elevated levels of cortisol can result in feelings of depression and anxiety.

Adrenaline, or epinephrine, is a neurotransmitter and hormone that basically does everything it can to raise your blood sugar and keep it elevated. Adrenaline inhibits insulin secretion, promotes the secretion of glucagon by the pancreas, stimulates glycogenolysis in the liver and muscles, stimulates glycolysis in the muscles, and increases heart rate and blood pressure. Over time, chronic elevation of this stress hormone can cause the following issues:

- Anxiety
- Depression
- Digestive problems
- Headaches
- Heart disease
- Memory and concentration impairment
- Sleep problems
- Weight gain

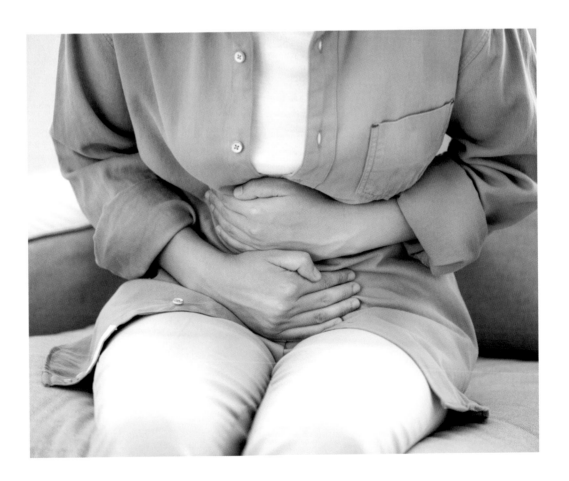

According to Volek and Phinney, adequate salt intake can prevent these issues. But because the keto diet makes sodium deficiency a high likelihood due to fast excretion, and many keto dieters don't get their sodium checked, the potential risk from long-term ketogenic dieting is something to seriously consider.

Aside from the health problems that stem from imbalances in sodium, potassium, and cortisol, from a body composition standpoint, elevated cortisol makes muscle gains extremely difficult to achieve. Because cortisol is catabolic, it breaks down molecules and inhibits muscle protein synthesis.

Lack of quality sleep from elevated cortisol and adrenaline will further prevent you from building muscle. Your body produces muscle-building hormones—including human growth hormone (HGH), which helps you build muscle mass and boosts metabolism—while you sleep. When your brain reaches the REM phase of sleep, your body heals and renews organs, tissues, and bones; regenerates immune cells; and stimulates HGH secretion.

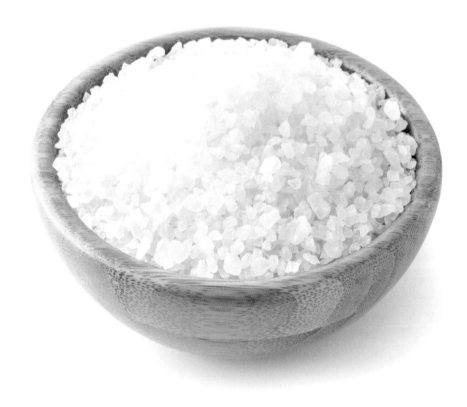

I'm not saying you can't build muscle on a ketogenic diet, but it's *easier* to slip into states of catabolic stress that prevent muscle growth. So, if building muscle is your goal, incorporating carbohydrates into your diet will help mitigate that risk.

In general, this propensity toward chronically elevated cortisol and adrenaline on a ketogenic diet because of the difficulty to maintain appropriate electrolyte balance is a reason I suggest reintroducing healthy carbohydrates after you've achieved the intended benefits of keto.

I recommend asking your doctor to check your levels or getting a hair mineral analysis (I use UpgradedFormulas.com with my clients). I have had clients with sky-high levels of sodium and potassium on keto and clients whose levels were too low. It's important to find out. And remember that if you are doing any extreme diet, you need to be prepared to monitor your vitals regularly.

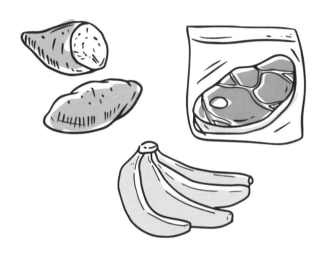

DOES THE BODY REALLY PREFER KETONES?

I find it interesting that in a ketogenic state, our bodies start doing things to increase available blood glucose. In my opinion, the body shows us over and over again that glucose is its preferred fuel source. Let's consider a few things:

- Your body turns extra protein into what? Glucose, not ketones.
- In a ketogenic state (unless you have the help of a research scientist telling you to eat more salt), your body elevates hormones that increase what? Glucose, not ketones.
- If you eat equal amounts of fat and carbs, your body runs on what? Glucose, not ketones.

I have never been able to wrap my head around the statement "the body prefers ketones." What?! No, it doesn't. This may be true if you're in a state of poor metabolism, but telling the general population that their bodies prefer ketones? That's just false. When given both carbs and fat, the body runs primarily on glucose. Even when a person is in a state of ketosis, portions of the brain must run on glucose. I believe nature leaves us clues, and the clues I'm seeing here are the body's way of saying, "I prefer to run on glucose, but I can also run on ketones." Interesting food for thought.

YOU MAY NOT BE ABLE TO SLEEP QUITE AS WELL

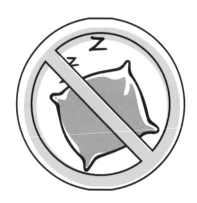

In addition to the potential of elevated cortisol and adrenaline preventing good-quality sleep on keto, there are some more considerations when it comes to sleep.

First, let me say that keto improves sleep for some people. These people tend to have high glutamate and low GABA. As mentioned earlier, glutamate is an excitatory neurotransmitter, whereas GABA is an inhibitory neurotransmitter. People with high glutamate and low GABA, therefore, may experience things like insomnia, mood swings, social anxiety, hypersensitivity, addiction, and racing thoughts. And since ketones increase the action of the GAD enzyme that helps convert glutamate to GABA, keto can help people with this issue feel calmer and think more clearly, and they often find it easier to sleep.

But that's not the case for everyone, specifically those with low serotonin. Energy, focus, calmness, ability to sleep, and a general sense of well-being are all dependent on healthy serotonin levels. Low serotonin causes anxiety, makes it more difficult to turn your brain off, and makes it more difficult to sleep. The absence of carbohydrates over long periods of time prevents the amino acid tryptophan from entering the brain, where it is converted to serotonin. If you eat carbs and protein, you'll favor tryptophan, increasing serotonin. If you eat protein and fats (keto), you'll produce more dopamine but much less serotonin.

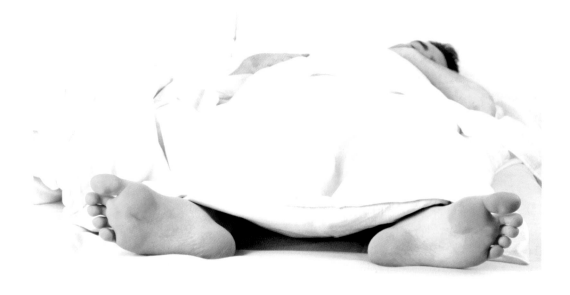

So, for people who don't have great serotonin levels to begin with, being on keto can cause them to become more anxious, lose motivation and focus, and have more difficulty sleeping.

From a body composition standpoint, there is nothing more crucial than adequate sleep. Sleep balances your mood, helps you make good food choices, promotes tissue healing and regeneration, and allows you to build muscle and more easily get the results you're after.

YOU MAY FEEL LESS SATISFIED AFTER MEALS AND BE PRONE TO OVEREATING OR BINGEING

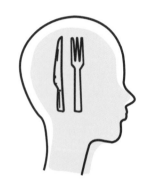

When I switched to keto, one of my biggest frustrations was that I never felt satisfied after meals. Everywhere I turned, people were talking about this amazing satiation benefit that they were getting from keto, while I would just sit there going, "Really?" I figured there was something wrong with me.

Yes, I could go a long time without eating and feel fine. However, when I did eat, I never felt satiated at the end of a meal. I had this unnerving feeling of dissatisfaction every time I finished eating. It often led me to the pantry for nuts, nut butter, pork rinds, or keto cookies in an attempt to find satisfaction. That never worked, and I ended up overconsuming calories—by a lot. It was so bad that sometimes I didn't even want to eat because I was afraid that once I opened the floodgates, I was never going to stop.

I tried so many things to mitigate it. I ate more slowly—like a lot more slowly—eating the same amount of food but prolonging each meal over the course of an hour. I stayed hydrated with salt, water, and other minerals. I ate tons of protein. Still, the same problem occurred the entire time I was keto, no matter what I did.

However, when I started bringing carbohydrates back in, I noticed right away that this issue was gone. If I could polish off some strawberries to my heart's content at the end of my meal, or maybe a sweet potato, or any whole-food carbohydrate, I felt satisfied and blissful, and I easily moved on.

As I reflected on this experience, I chalked it up to two things: insulin and fiber.

Insulin is often demonized as the "fat storage hormone" and something we want to avoid at all costs in the keto community, which is shortsighted. Insulin does transport excess energy to fat stores, and chronically high insulin levels are a sign of metabolic dysfunction for sure. However, insulin serves a lot of awesome purposes in the body, like shuttling energy into our cells and helping us feel full! Research shows that insulin sensitizes our brains to meal-generated satiety signals.[19]

On top of that, consider the fiber you get from carbs. A pound of strawberries, for example, has 9 grams of fiber (and only 145 calories, I might add). And because I know you're curious, those strawberries have 35 grams of carbs. Strawberries are about 60 percent insoluble fiber and 40 percent soluble fiber.

Soluble fiber pulls in and swells up with water in the stomach, partially dissolving within it to form a thick gel-like substance in the stomach that slows digestion. This is what tempers the blood sugar response, making carbohydrates with fiber "slower" carbs than a straight glucose source with no fiber. Insoluble fiber, on the other hand, doesn't dissolve; it remains intact in your stomach, further promoting volume and a feeling of fullness when you're eating.

So, when I eat some carbs with my meal, I have a full stomach, and I'm more sensitive to satiety signals from the insulin increase. Jackpot. Now I'm full and ready to move on from the meal.

Here's my take on why I think a small increase in carbohydrates (around 100 to 150 grams per day total) pretty effortlessly helped me drop 7 pounds of fat and build 8 pounds of muscle:

If I can feel full and satisfied from 145 calories' worth of strawberries and maintain a healthy blood sugar response, that's going to be more beneficial for long-term weight management than chronically digging into the nut butter jar and downing 600 calories before I know what happened. On top of that, because I'm very active and not overeating, those 35 grams of carbohydrates will likely be stored as muscle glycogen, fueling athletic performance in my next workout and creating a favorable internal environment for insulin sensitivity, muscle growth, and healthy body composition long term.

I have to add that even though folks on the internet often talk about how they're never hungry on keto, I can't tell you how many people I have worked with one-on-one have revealed that they have bingeing issues on keto. If they're not full-on bingeing, they still have a lot of pantry-raiding overeating sessions. And often, those overeating sessions involve the worst kinds of carbs, leaving them feeling like crap the next day. When they allow themselves to eat a balanced diet again, these issues go away. This evidence is anecdotal, of course, but I would love to see some sort of scientific report on it because in my experience, it is extremely common among keto dieters.

BENEFITS OF CARBOHYDRATES AND
WHY YOU MIGHT CONSIDER THEM AFTER A KETO PHASE

So maybe you're on a ketogenic diet and you're reading this, thinking, "I stay on top of my salt intake, I sleep fine, and I don't have any problems with satiation. I feel like a million bucks on keto. It's the best I've ever felt. I love this lifestyle."

Do I still think you should bring carbs back in? My advice is always this: if you are truly thriving, keep doing your thing. Do you feel incredible? Is everything going amazingly well? Your labs are good, your mood is good, your sleep is good, and you've reached (or are getting close to reaching) your body goals? I say keep going.

If you are using keto as a therapeutic tool to heal something like epilepsy, cancer, or type 2 diabetes, I will be very honest: I don't know when, or if, you should bring carbs back in. I will leave it to my colleagues who specialize in the therapeutic applications of a ketogenic diet to help you with that. If you are looking for trusted resources, I recommend visiting the website MetabolicHealthSummit.com and/or attending one of their events. That is where I find the latest research from the medical communities involved in therapeutic applications of keto. LowCarbUSA.com is also a wonderful resource, presenting lots of evidence-based research.

But, if you are using keto as a health optimization tool, there are a few points I'd like you to consider.

We hear so many horrible things about carbohydrates in the keto world, and I'm afraid we have forgotten the beauty of creation that is the carbohydrate. They are little gifts from nature that give us life. And they share an incredible relationship with us human beings as well as all other life forms. They are intrinsic to our survival. When we look at them for what they are in the natural cycle—wow, they are amazing. And amazing for us.

Let's break down the word:

Carbo = carbon

Hydrate = water

Carbohydrates are simply carbon and water.

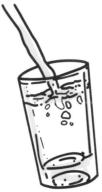

You know how we get calories, or energy, from carbohydrates? Plants make glucose, or energy, *out of thin air,* literally. Plants are considered producers because they produce their own glucose without the need for eating. We humans are considered consumers because we rely on eating for energy. It's hard for us to wrap our heads around this concept as consumers, but plants make glucose out of water, air, and light. Respect, right? That's pretty cool.

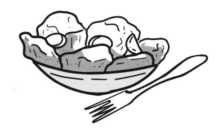

And let me be more specific: plants make glucose, or energy, out of water, light, and *carbon dioxide,* the very thing we humans breathe out and give to them. In addition to glucose, plants produce oxygen for us to breathe in. It's a mutual relationship of give and take; plants need us, and we need them.

Of course, it's not just about glucose and oxygen. Plants also deliver the vital vitamins, minerals, phytonutrients, carotenoids, bioflavonoids, and polyphenols that we need to survive. We can get most (but not all) of those things from animals. So why do we want the glucose when we can just eat meat and make ketones?

- Your brain, organs, and blood do need some glucose, even in a ketogenic state. Your body will be forced to make its own glucose if you don't eat any. It does so by taking amino acids from the protein you eat (or by breaking down your muscle tissue into amino acids) to make glucose through a process called gluconeogenesis. Don't you think it would be easier to just eat a little glucose than to constantly make your body do it the hard way?

- When you have adequate levels of stored muscle glycogen, you are better able to exercise at high intensities. This, in turn, makes you more insulin sensitive, and you develop higher levels of HGH, making muscle-building and fat-burning easier.

- You prevent the risk of chronically elevated cortisol and adrenaline.

- You prevent the risk of chronically low serotonin.

- You protect your gut lining by feeding nondigestible fiber to the bacteria in your colon, whose metabolites (short-chain fatty acids) exert positive effects on the intestinal mucosa. The lack of these metabolites has been found to cause the bacteria to feed on the mucosal lining itself, resulting in leaky gut, a condition in which the gut lining has tiny gaps that allow bacteria and toxins to flow into the bloodstream.

In a nutshell, a diet that includes healthy carbohydrates from nature makes it easier for us to be healthy, fit, and thriving.

Here are some signs that you and your body might be ready to bring carbs back:

- You just aren't feeling that great anymore on keto.
- You're not getting the results you want, no matter what you do.
- You're losing muscle and/or gaining fat on keto.
- You have developed an unhealthy relationship with food, finding yourself in a restrict-and-binge cycle, for example.
- You're not sleeping well.
- You've had a gradual increase in anxiety since starting keto.
- You have a general sense of unhappiness on keto.
- Your exercise performance still sucks, and you've given keto at least several months.
- You're overeating because you don't feel satisfied at the ends of your meals.
- You have healthy blood sugar regulation and have no real reason not to eat carbs.
- You're not eating carbs purely because deep down you're afraid you'll get fat if you do.
- You have chronic watery stools or constipation on keto, no matter what you do.
- When you do eat carbs, you eat all the unhealthy ones because "it's now or never."

The answer to how long you should do keto is incredibly individual. However, in general, you can use this list and also look at it in this simple way: the higher your body fat percentage, fasting blood sugar, and inflammation markers and the lower your activity level, the longer you will benefit from keto.

Once you have stopped losing weight on keto, your fasted morning blood sugar is under 90, and you are not using keto to heal anything in your body, I recommend reintroducing carbohydrates as I show you how to do in the meal plan in Appendix C. It's ideal to match the meal plan to the training plan I have provided or to your own workout schedule so that you use the carbs you eat and also continue increasing insulin sensitivity through exercise.

Increasing carbohydrates after keto is an exploratory time during which I recommend paying close attention to how your body is responding. Pay attention to your exercise performance, sleep, satiety, digestion, and mood—and definitely to your relationship with food. This is a tricky issue for many keto dieters, so let's dive into restoring your emotional relationship with carbohydrates after keto.

IS THERE A "RIGHT" AMOUNT OF TIME FOR KETO?

There's no standard length of time to do keto. I do recommend most people do it for one to six months to really allow the adaptation to occur and find out how your body does once it's fully keto adapted. I highly recommend you push that toward the six-month end of the range, as the body will run more efficiently on ketones over time. But if you are into your keto journey and feel really horrible, you've hired a coach or have heavily researched how to optimize things and you still feel like garbage, by all means, there's no trophy for making it to six months. Take care of yourself and do what feels right to you. But do remember that most people don't feel awesome right away on keto, especially in the first week or two—it takes time.

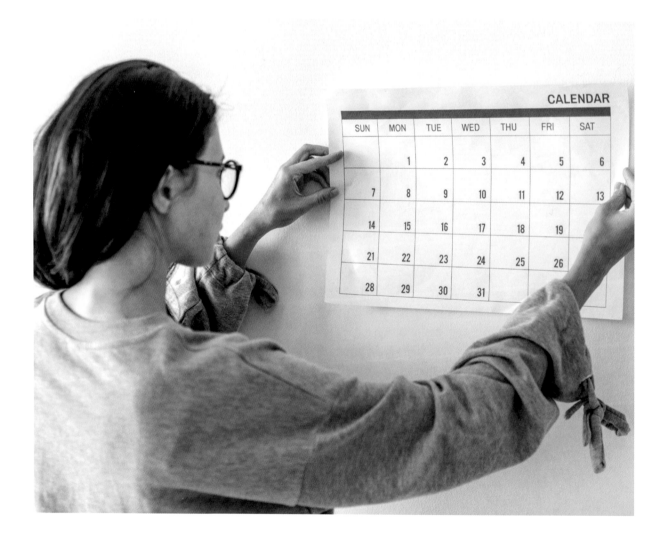

RESTORING YOUR RELATIONSHIP WITH CARBOHYDRATES

Through working with people over the years, I've found that some won't let go of keto even though it often isn't working well for them anymore. This is especially common in people who achieved significant weight loss with keto but are now getting negative health results. They're anxious, losing their hair, not making physical progress—they're honestly kind of a wreck. However, because they've developed a deep belief that keto is optimal, they keep going. But when we bring carbohydrates back in, they become calm, confident, and start getting results again.

I have found that the thing that holds most people back from reintroducing carbohydrates is fear. They are afraid they'll be hungry all the time, gain weight, go back to "how they used to be," and totally lose control.

Allow me to share a story from one of my wonderful clients, Despina, who had lost over 100 pounds on keto and came to me for help losing the last 5 to 15 pounds she wanted to shed. These are her words:

> In 2018, after giving up on myself after becoming a mom, I got my act together, got my nutrition together, started working on my mindset, and started moving my body. And I started keto. I wasn't even a strict keto-er in that I tracked net carbs, stayed around 20 to 25 grams net per day, and still ate some vegetables and fruit.
>
> It worked. I lost 96 pounds in the first six months. I then spent the next twelve months losing an additional 25 pounds and falling in love with working out along the way.
>
> As you can imagine, I felt AMAZING...until I didn't. Until my energy started suffering. My workouts weren't good. I could not sleep, and I was up at 4 a.m. each day—not in a good way but in a jittery, fight-or-flight type of energy way. I also started experiencing hair loss. And no matter what I did, those last 5 to 15 pounds I wanted to shed would. not. come. off!
>
> This little voice in my head was telling me: you need to change something. And that something might be adding in some carbs, especially around workouts. My protein was probably too low, too, as I was following more traditional keto macros. But I was so in love with this way of eating that had gotten me the kind of results that I'd never gotten before, having struggled with weight my whole life. So, instead of leaning into that intuitive whisper, I dug deeper into keto.

I researched other ways of eating, followed all the big fitness and nutrition influencers on social media, read everything I could get my hands on...and the keto people all seemed to have the same message. Stick it out. Carbs are bad. Maybe even try carnivore to see if what you have is a sensitivity to something. Like maybe you aren't keto enough!

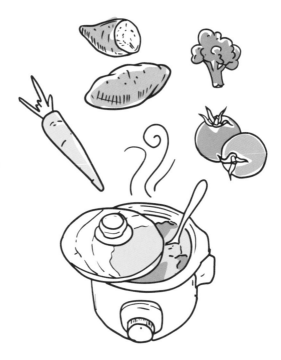

Enter Tara. I'd followed her on social media for a while, and I listened when she talked about going in and out of ketosis and being metabolically flexible. And I thought, well, that works for other people—healthy people—who haven't been as overweight as I have been. It won't work for me.

But, in desperation, I tried on my own to add in some carbs. And you know what happened? I went off the rails. Having some carbs, my body was like YES, PLEASE—MORE. But it wasn't just physical; it was also that I'd made carbs the enemy. So once I had some of this very bad, forbidden thing and failed, I just threw all my hard work away and totally overate them.

I kept trying and was stuck in this bad cycle. Then I'd restrict the carbs and get back to "normal," lose those extra few pounds again...except I couldn't sustain my old keto normal. I didn't feel good. I wasn't satisfied. I was increasing the intensity of my workouts and wanted to feel strong, but I kept feeling spent.

So I contacted Tara and started working with her individually. We went through all of my health history, nutrition, macros, bloodwork, DNA testing...all of it. She put an insane amount of thought into every single recommendation she made for me—both on a physical level with food and vitamin recommendations and workouts, but also on a spiritual level—like this is the deep work you need to do to continue on this journey of transformation. And that plan included, you guessed it, bringing carbs back in—not pizza and donuts, but sweet potatoes and veggies to my heart's desire, especially on training days.

You can guess what happened. I actually started healing my relationship with food. My workouts started improving. You could see my muscles as I was getting strong and leaner at the same time! My sleep improved. My heart rate variability improved (Tara also monitored my Oura ring data).

This journey is never-ending. We are all perpetual students. But working with Tara gave me tools that I use every day. She set me on a path to doing deep, personal development work without which I don't think I could have continued on this path. The statistics are pretty terrible for how many people lose weight and actually keep the weight off. But, with all the mind, body, and spirit tools I took away from our working together, I know deep in my soul that it isn't something I have to worry about anymore. This is who I am. Forever grateful for her, and we are all so lucky that she is doing this work and sharing her knowledge. Her social media and podcasts teach me, re-center me, and re-motivate me to better myself every day!

And her message—do a phase of keto, learn about nutrition, heal your body, and teach it to be metabolically flexible, and then, if you aren't feeling so good, add some whole food–based carbs back in to see how your body responds—SO MANY NEED TO HEAR THIS. Keto is amazing! And I still have days that are more keto than low carb. But when I'm training hard or if I'm just needing nutrients, I eat nutrient-dense carbs and feel amazing!

I'm so proud of Despina, and I share her story because this scenario is becoming very typical; I've coached so many people who are in a similar place. Keto served its purpose, but people who've done keto for a while start not to feel so good anymore. They stop getting results while having a fear-based relationship with *all* carbohydrates, even healthy ones. This woman had perfect blood sugar by the time she came to me; she wasn't in the same body that she had been in when she started her keto journey. She was extremely fit and active by this point. She was doing high-intensity interval training. I knew carbs would not only help her get results by supporting her capacity to perform optimally in the anaerobic states in which she was training, but would also

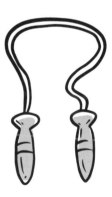

help her sleep and recover, further promoting results, not to mention reducing her anxiety.

Here's another point that I think is interesting. This woman was a type 3 in the Neurotyping System created by Christian Thibaudeau (thibarmy.com), who has mentored me on this system that I've been using with my clients for several years with great success. The Neurotyping System is based on a personality test that Thibaudeau designed with his parents, both psychologists, using personality traits as clues to a person's neurotransmitter levels. The type 3 "neurotype" tends to have higher glutamate, lower GABA, and higher cortisol and adrenaline. Thibaudeau describes the type 3 as a catch-22, because if the person has had high cortisol for many years, they can become insulin resistant, but they also need carbs more than any other type to help prevent the rise of cortisol and adrenaline to which they are prone.

I typically take my type 3 clients through a phase of keto to restore insulin sensitivity and healthy blood sugar regulation, as I've found that quite often they do have insulin resistance. Once their blood sugar regulation is healthy, we reintroduce carbs, and this is pretty much always the result: their stress levels go down, they start sleeping better, and they start getting better body composition results. Exercise performance increases, and so does their ability to recover from those workouts—all with normal cortisol levels that come as a result of healthy blood sugar regulation and regular carbohydrate consumption.

If you are fearful of bringing carbohydrates back in, I recommend starting very slowly and experimenting with small amounts. Add some strawberries to your salad. Have a sweet potato with dinner. Healthy carbohydrates shouldn't make you feel any different. In fact, they should make you feel pretty amazing.

And if eating a sweet potato leads you into a carbohydrate frenzy, please keep in mind that this is quite possibly a sign of a disordered relationship with food, not because you went out of ketosis and had some physiological trigger. I discuss this further in Chapter 3.

Many people who are still keto, or coming off keto, think they have a carb addiction, when in reality, they just have a restrictive mindset around carbs. It is this mindset that causes them to eat "all the carbs" if they eat even one carb. This is common with any type of extreme dietary restriction. Bikini competitors are notorious for doing it with peanut butter. They don't have a "peanut butter addiction"; it's just the one calorically dense food they're "allowed" to have on their extreme calorie-restricted diet. And sometimes when they are super stressed, they have one spoonful and then can't stop, and find themselves bingeing on it.

If this sort of thing is happening to you, you may want to reach out to a specialist who helps with disordered eating. A tendency to binge may be all the more reason to restore your relationship with carbohydrates and reintroduce them into your diet. Being healthy, fit, and thriving doesn't have to be super restrictive. Life doesn't have to be that way.

As a coach, one of my biggest concerns about the ketogenic diet is a restrictive mindset around food. All you read online is that keto curbs cravings and you no longer want sugar or carbs. But in working with people one-on-one, I have found this to be rare. More often, clients come to me with extremely poor relationships with food as a result of keto. (I find it more common in women than men, but it does affect men, too.) I am, quite frankly, concerned. If you fall into this category, please consider slowly reintroducing a small amount of healthy carbohydrates into your diet, and hire a coach to help you through the process if you need to.

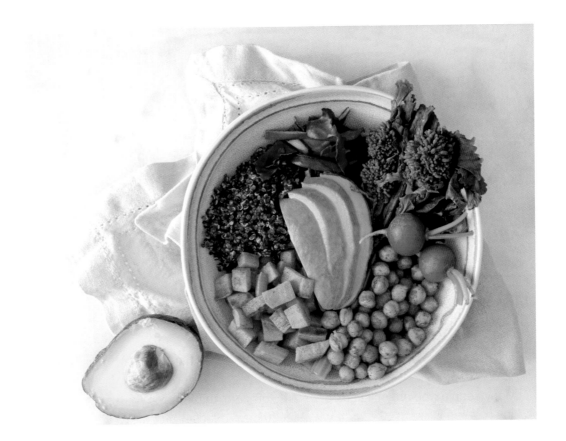

BIOFEEDBACK TO LOOK FOR
WHILE REINTRODUCING CARBOHYDRATES

My biggest concern for clients who reintroduce carbohydrates is digestion. Please remember that, just like when you switched to keto and it took your body a little while to produce adequate enzymes to digest all that fat, it's going to take your body some time to realize that it needs to upregulate amylase to help you digest more carbs.

Some bloating and irregular bowel movements are to be expected, especially because you are increasing your fiber intake. You can help offset these effects by taking digestive enzymes during the transition. I recommend a digestive enzyme complex that contains amylase as well as betaine HCl, which increases stomach acid and helps you break down your food to absorb more nutrients. Be mindful to take it in the middle of your meals, because if you increase stomach acid on an empty stomach, you may throw up. If, after a week or two, you are still experiencing a lot of bloating from particular carbohydrates, I recommend taking a break from those foods and eating ones that you tolerate better.

Also make sure to stay hydrated to help with gut motility.

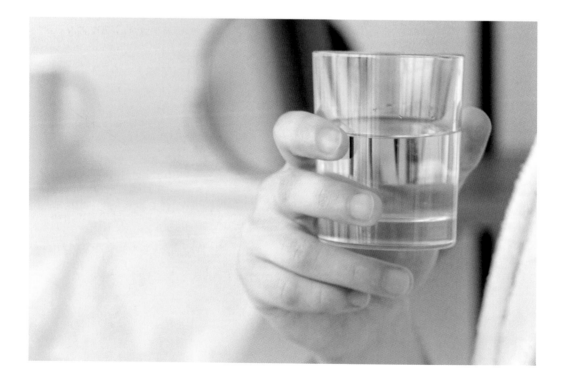

Here are some other effects you may notice:

- **You will gain a few pounds of scale weight right off the bat.** This is water! Please expect this and don't let it deter you. Our psychotic relationship with scale numbers is mind-boggling sometimes. You will retain approximately 3 grams of water for every 1 gram of carbohydrates eaten. That means if you eat 100 grams of carbs, you can expect to hold on to 300 grams of water. You might actually look better depending on how lean you are and how much muscle you have. (See my next point.)

- **Your muscles will look fuller.** Depending on how many carbs you incorporate, water will be drawn into your muscles as your muscle glycogen refills, leaving you looking leaner and more muscular.

- **Your energy in workouts will likely go up.** Enjoy!

- **You should feel just as good as you did on keto.** If you're incorporating healthy carbohydrates from nature, you should feel fantastic. This will not be the case if you choose cake and ice cream as your carbohydrate sources.

- **If you notice an increase in joint aches or muscle soreness, try different carbohydrate sources and troubleshoot.** You could have sensitivities to certain foods.

If you can afford it, I highly recommend getting a continuous glucose monitor (CGM) to use during this phase of your journey. I wore one and it blew my mind how different my blood sugar response was to foods than all the textbooks say it "should" be. This is often the case! You may find that bananas barely make your blood sugar budge, whereas strawberries make it spike. It could be the opposite for someone else. We are learning that the blood sugar response to different foods is more bioindividual than previously known. If you can't afford a continuous glucose monitor, you can get a blood glucose monitor and check yourself every thirty minutes for up to four hours after eating to study your blood sugar response to a particular food or meal.

In the next chapter, I dive deeper into what you can expect as you reintroduce carbohydrates, issues to be aware of, how to best mitigate them, which are the best kinds of carbs to choose, when to most intelligently eat them, and how you can expect them to affect you.

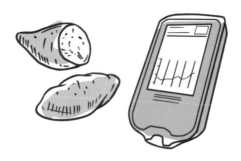

REFERENCES

1. Karen Hardy et al., "The Importance of Dietary Carbohydrate in Human Evolution," *The Quarterly Review of Biology* 90, no. 3 (2015): 251–68, https://doi.org/10.1086/682587.

2. Pim Knuiman, Maria T. E. Hopman, and Marco Mensink, "Glycogen Availability and Skeletal Muscle Adaptations with Endurance and Resistance Exercise," *Nutrition & Metabolism* 12 (2015), accessed June 27, 2021, https://doi.org/10.1186/s12986-015-0055-9.

3. Craig Freudenrich, "How Fat Cells Work," HowStuffWorks, accessed June 27, 2021, https://science.howstuffworks.com/life/cellular-microscopic/fat-cell2.htm.

4. John C. Newman and Eric Verdin, "ß-Hydroxybutyrate: Much More Than a Metabolite," *Diabetes Research and Clinical Practice* 106, no. 2 (2014): 173–81, https://doi.org/10.1016/j.diabres.2014.08.009.

5. Gregory A. Nichols, Teresa A. Hillier, and Jonathan B. Brown, "Normal Fasting Plasma Glucose and Risk of Type 2 Diabetes Diagnosis," *American Journal of Medicine* 121, no. 6 (2008): 519–21, https://doi.org/10.1016/j.amjmed.2008.02.026, https://www.amjmed.com/article/S0002-9343(08)00231-3/fulltext.

6. Guido Freckmann et al., "Continuous Glucose Profiles in Healthy Subjects Under Everyday Life Conditions and After Different Meals," *Journal of Diabetes Science and Technology* 1, no. 5 (2007): 695–703, https://doi.org/10.1177/193229680700100513.

7. Robert J. Adams et al., "Independent Association of HbA(1c) and Incident Cardiovascular Disease in People Without Diabetes," *Obesity* 17, no. 3 (2009): 559–63, https://doi.org/10.1038/oby.2008.592.

8. Kimberly P. Kinzig, Mary A. Honors, and Sara L. Hargrave, "Insulin Sensitivity and Glucose Tolerance Are Altered by Maintenance on a Ketogenic Diet," *Endocrinology* 151, no. 7 (2010): 3105–14, https://doi.org/10.1210/en.2010-0175.

9. Cleveland Clinic, "Fat: What You Need to Know," accessed June 27, 2021, https://my.clevelandclinic.org/health/articles/11208-fat-what-you-need-to-know.

10. Chrysi Koliaki et al., "The Effect of Ingested Macronutrients on Postprandial Ghrelin Response: A Critical Review of Existing Literature Data," *International Journal of Peptides* 2010, accessed June 27, 2021, https://doi.org/10.1155/2010/710852.

11. Stephen C. Benoit et al., "Palmitic Acid Mediates Hypothalamic Insulin Resistance by Altering PKC-Theta Subcellular Localization in Rodents," *Journal of Clinical Investigation* 119, no. 9 (2009): 2577–89, https://doi.org/10.1172/JCI36714.

12. Laura C. Ortinau et al., "Effects of High-Protein vs. High- Fat Snacks on Appetite Control, Satiety, and Eating Initiation in Healthy Women," *Nutrition Journal* 13, no. 1 (2014), accessed June 27, 2021, https://doi.org/10.1186/1475-2891-13-97.

13. Mark Hyman, "Slow Carbs, Not Low Carbs: The Truth About Low-Carb Diets," Dr. Hyman, accessed June 27, 2021, https://drhyman.com/blog/2015/08/20/slow-carbs-not-low-carbs-the-truth-about-low-carb-diets/.

14. Adam L. Hartman et al., "The Neuropharmacology of the Ketogenic Diet," *Pediatric Neurology* 36, no. 5 (2007): 281–92, https://doi.org/10.1016/j.pediatrneurol.2007.02.008.

15. Sharmineh Sharafi and Leila Nateghi, "Optimization of Gamma-Aminobutyric Acid Production by Probiotic Bacteria Through Response Surface Methodology," *Iranian Journal of Microbiology* 12, no. 6 (2020): 581–91, https://doi.org/10.18502/ijm.v12i6.5033.

16. William H. Church, Ryan E. Adams, and Livia S. Wyss, "Ketogenic Diet Alters Dopaminergic Activity in the Mouse Cortex," *Neuroscience Letters* 571 (2014): 1–4, https://doi.org/10.1016/j.neulet.2014.04.016.

17. See note 5 above.

18. Stephen Phinney and Jeff Volek, "Sodium, Nutritional Ketosis, and Adrenal Function," Virta Health, accessed June 27, 2021, https://www.virtahealth.com/blog/sodium-nutritional-ketosis-keto-flu-adrenal-function.

19. See note 6 above.

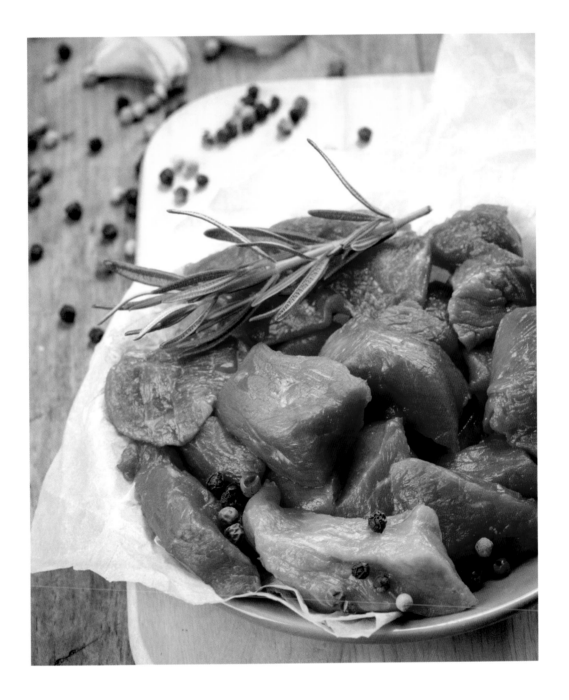

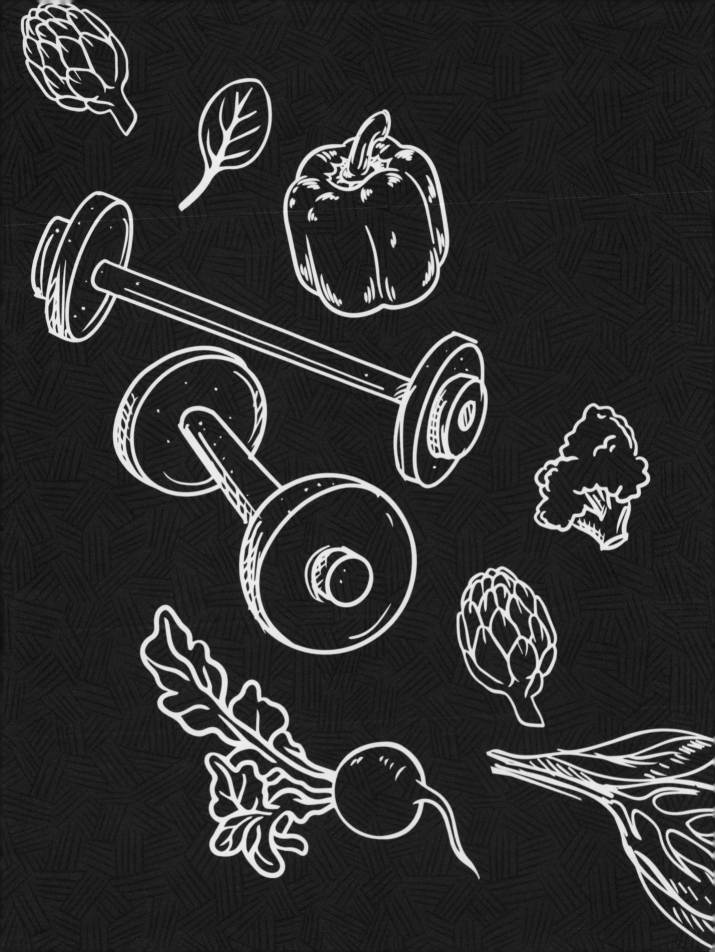

CHAPTER 3

HOW TO BRING CARBS BACK IN AND MATCH YOUR WORKOUTS WITH YOUR NUTRITION

The biggest question I get in regard to bringing carbs back in is, "How many carbs should I eat?" Before I jump into the numbers, I want to address an even more important issue: the *types* of carbs you'll want to prioritize as you fill out those numbers.

As we know, carbs are currently blamed for being the culprit in obesity and diabetes. But is that really the truth? Are carbohydrates the problem? Or are *processed* carbohydrates the problem? Let's take a look.

The healthiest populations in the world eat carbs. People in Hong Kong and Japan have the longest life spans, and carbs are the backbone of both of their diets. We can learn from them and other populations who eat high-carbohydrate diets and enjoy longevity and high quality of life that the problem is not carbohydrates. The problem is the *types* and *amounts* of carbohydrates—and calories in general—that people are eating.

What does the typical diet in Hong Kong consist of? Mostly fish, fruits, vegetables, rice, nut oils, and meat. Carbs, yes. But what kinds of carbs? Minimally processed carbs from nature.

What about Japan? The Japanese diet revolves around rice, fresh vegetables, pickled vegetables, fish, and fermented soy products. In Okinawa, specifically, a "Blue Zone" where the highest percentage of centenarians (people who live to be 100 years old or older) in the world reside, the sweet potato is a dietary staple. Until recent years, the Okinawan diet consisted of *85 percent carbohydrates!* That number has dropped to about 60 percent as people have begun eating more protein and fat, but it is still a high-carbohydrate diet.[1]

It is notable that these populations are eating high-carbohydrate, low-fat diets that prioritize whole, unprocessed carbohydrates from nature...and they're living longer than the rest of us.

Let's talk about rice for a second. I love talking about rice, which is such a no-no in the low-carb world. But let's take a look:

China consumes more rice than any other country in the world. The obesity rate in China is 5 to 6 percent, which is higher than it might be only because of the higher obesity rates in cities where American fast food is popular, which reach 20 percent or higher.

Meanwhile, the obesity rate in the United States is 42.4 percent and climbing. And we sit over here pointing the finger at rice, singling it out as if it was the problem.

Another example is the bodybuilding community. White rice is a staple food for bodybuilders, who reach some of the lowest body fat percentages in the world.

The problem is not rice. The problem is not carbohydrates from nature. The problems are eating too many processed carbs, reduced physical activity, and overeating.

In Okinawa, the practice of not overeating is embedded into the culture. Okinawans live by the principle of hara hachi bu, a Confucian teaching that instructs people to eat until they are 80 percent full. Bodybuilders also practice caloric restriction.

So what can we learn here?

- Clearly, carbohydrates are not generally "bad for you" if, in the place where the most people on Earth live to be 100, people are eating a diet that's 60 to 85 percent carbs.

- Clearly, carbohydrates do not singlehandedly "make you fat" if the leanest people in the world eat an abundance of them.

- The types of carbs people are eating make a huge difference.

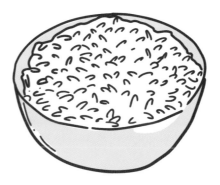

Under the current American paradigm, a carb is a carb. The general message people are receiving from low-carb advocates is: just don't eat carbs. French fries, apples, chocolate donuts, quinoa—they're all the same, and they all need to go if you want to be healthier and lose weight. This thinking is painfully shortsighted. Eating the *right kinds* of carbohydrates can actually make fat loss easier and improve overall health.

So let's dive into the different types of carbs. I'm putting these in order of priority for making fat loss and weight maintenance easier, but that doesn't necessarily mean you should avoid the ones that fall lower on the list. It just means that if you tend to fill up on the ones I've rated higher, you will have an easier time maintaining your weight over the long term.

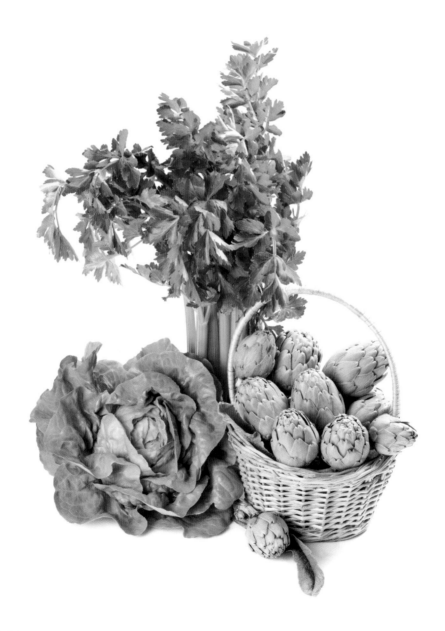

CARB SOURCE PRIORITY #1:
NONSTARCHY VEGETABLES

I know you've heard this advice before, but it's the truth: eat your veggies.

The number one type of carb that you'll want to fill up on is nonstarchy vegetables. If you do this, everything will get easier. Nonstarchy vegetables include

- Artichokes
- Asparagus
- Bean sprouts
- Broccoli
- Brussels sprouts
- Cabbage
- Cauliflower
- Celery
- Cucumbers
- Eggplant
- Leafy greens
- Mushrooms
- Onions
- Peppers
- Spinach
- Summer squash, such as yellow squash and zucchini
- Tomatoes
- Turnips

Why are nonstarchy vegetables so important? They have two qualities that make them the stars of the show when it comes to healthy body weight and overall health:

- **They pack in nutrition for very few calories.** You get a lot of bang for your buck calorically.
- **They fill you up and keep you full.** Vegetables are loaded with fiber. Fiber will fill you up at mealtime, slow your blood sugar response and keep it from going too high, build healthy gut bacteria, and delay gastric emptying so you stay fuller longer.

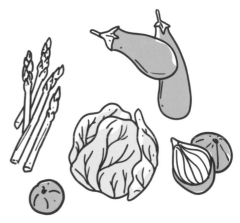

CARB SOURCE PRIORITY #2: STARCHY VEGETABLES

Next on the list in terms of priority and quantity of carbohydrates is starchy vegetables:

- Beans, such as chickpeas, kidney beans, and lima beans
- Beets
- Carrots
- Corn
- Lentils
- Parsnips
- Peas
- Potatoes
- Pumpkin
- Sweet potatoes
- Taro
- Winter squash, such as acorn or butternut
- Yams

Starchy vegetables generally have a higher carbohydrate content than nonstarchy vegetables, so you can think of them as energy powerhouses. They will fill up your glycogen tanks faster, providing you with sustained energy. Just be careful not to overindulge in them, or the extra glucose can spill over into your fat stores.

In terms of blood sugar response, starchy vegetables will create a higher level than nonstarchy vegetables will. However, please remember that having a blood sugar rise from food is normal; it is not a concern when your body can naturally restore your blood sugar to a healthy level. Also remember that starchy vegetables are rich sources of fiber, which slows the blood sugar response and helps with long-term healthy blood sugar levels.

This is where a continuous glucose monitor, which I recommended in the previous chapter (see page 79), will come in handy; it allows you to see your personal blood sugar response to foods. This response is extremely individual from person to person. Your gut microbiome, body composition, food sensitivities, activity level, and genetics all play into how you respond to carbohydrates.[2]

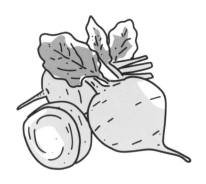

A note on beans: sometimes I get a shocked response on social media when I share recipes that include beans. Beans and other legumes get a bad rap in some health communities and are even prohibited on certain diets. There are lots of fears around the lectins and phytic acid in legumes because these antinutrients are believed to cause nutrient deficiencies and poor gut health.

While some people may be extremely sensitive to these compounds, most of us don't need to worry. Cooking and soaking beans has been shown to render lectins inactive. Also, if you have healthy gut bacteria, your body can break down phytic acid relatively easily. Ounce for ounce, there is more phytic acid in spinach, Swiss chard, walnuts, and almonds than in legumes. When we look at the overall picture, legumes are incredible sources of carbohydrates and fiber, they are full of vitamins and minerals, and they should be omitted only if someone has a unique biological sensitivity to them.

White potatoes have also been demonized for quite some time, as people are often afraid of blood sugar spikes from eating them. However, potatoes are full of potassium, vitamin C, vitamin B6, fiber, and many other vitamins and minerals. If you have healthy blood sugar regulation, your body can restore healthy blood sugar levels after a meal without a crash.

Also, keep in mind that you will normally eat potatoes with protein and fat, which will slow the blood sugar response. And if you boil and then cool your potatoes, they become resistant starch, which can actually lower your blood sugar levels.

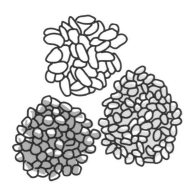

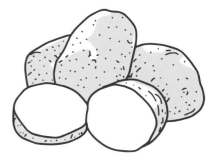

CARB SOURCE PRIORITY #3:
FRUITS

I'm talking whole, unprocessed fruits, especially if they are in season. Most people worry that fruit might be too high in sugar. However, even on the glycemic index (which some health communities now question because foods are tested in isolation, not eaten alongside other foods as they normally would be), most fruits have a low to medium impact when it comes to raising blood sugar.

Fruit is also chock-full of antioxidants, vitamins, and minerals, and it's a decent source of fiber. However, many people, especially in the low-carb community, fear eating fruit because of its fructose content, so let's talk about how fructose is processed in the body.

Nonstarchy vegetables (listed on page 87) are mostly glucose. Fruit, on the other hand, is mostly fructose, another type of sugar.

Once fructose is metabolized in your body, it is, by and large, equal to glucose since your liver turns it into glucose. From there, glucose goes straight from your gut into your bloodstream and is ready to be taken up by your cells, including your muscle cells and your liver, for energy. This is why I put starchy vegetables in the number two spot in this list. I want you to be able to fuel your cells and muscles efficiently with glucose, which is called glycogen once it is stored in your muscles and liver. When your muscles and liver are full of glycogen, any excess is stored as body fat.

So, in the end, both fructose and glucose end up as glucose and are converted to body fat only when the glycogen stores in your liver and muscles are completely full.

The liver can store approximately 80 to 100 grams of glycogen at a time. As long as you are not overdoing it and you are moving your body to use up that amount, you can look at fruit as an energy source without fearing that it will make you fat.

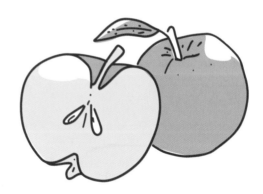

CARB SOURCE PRIORITY #4:
WHOLE GRAINS

I can practically hear my crucifixion being planned in the low-carb/keto/Paleo/ primal communities as I write this, but whole grains can actually improve blood sugar regulation.

A large study published in the *Journal of Nutrition* in 2018 looked at 55,465 people between the ages of fifty and sixty-five. The researchers found that the highest whole-grain intake among the male participants was associated with a 34 percent decreased risk of type 2 diabetes; the female participants who ate the most whole grains saw a 22 percent decreased risk.[3]

In Sardinia, Italy, another one of the world's "Blue Zones," people eat a diet that is 47 percent whole grains, mostly from—you ready for it?—bread. They also eat cheese and drink wine. Jealous? The classic Sardinian diet consists of whole-grain bread, beans, garden vegetables, and fruits. Meat is mostly reserved for Sundays and special occasions. But perhaps the key to this population's longevity is the high priority given to family, friends, laughing, and walking (something to consider as we scramble around in our fast-paced lives doing every diet trend in the book, stressed to the max and barely moving!). Their food is almost completely locally grown, which brings me to my next point.

When choosing whole grains, prioritize those that are organic and as close to their natural form as possible. Grains that are near to their natural form have more fiber, keeping your blood sugar stable and keeping you fuller longer. Locally grown organic grains are ideal. You do not want grains that have been genetically modified (the label will say non-GMO).

If you want to go the bread route, I recommend sourdough, or, if you want to make bread at home, you can order wheat flour from Italy online and see if you tolerate it better (try a tiny amount). Many people handle gluten-containing foods from Europe better than those made in the United States because grains grown in Europe generally haven't been genetically modified or treated with glyphosate, a toxic pesticide.

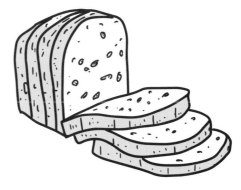

A note on grains: some people do have sensitivities to grains, so if you are experiencing digestive issues and/or achy joints, please see your doctor or naturopath for a healing protocol. Not everyone has issues with grains, though. The brainwashing that exists on this topic does not have sufficient scientific evidence to back it up, and it can potentially hold people's health back by instilling unwarranted fears. If you do not have any noticeable sensitivities to grains, they can be a tremendous source of nutrients in your diet.

Whole grains are excellent sources of fiber, vitamins, and minerals and include

- Amaranth
- Barley
- Brown rice
- Buckwheat (also a complete protein!)
- Bulgur wheat
- Farro
- Oats (steel-cut oats, rolled oats, oat groats)

- Popcorn
- Quinoa (also a complete protein!)
- Rye
- Spelt
- Wheat

While I encourage you to choose whole, unprocessed grains, remember that having an occasional piece of delicious bread is not going to do you in, especially if you are active. I personally don't eat a lot of bread, but rice, oats, and quinoa are regular parts of my diet.

In summary, when it comes to carbohydrate sources, I recommend nonstarchy and starchy vegetables first because they are generally less calorie dense and contain fewer carbohydrates, so you can indulge a little more. In our food-abundant world, it's extremely helpful to fill up on healthy foods that have fewer calories. For example:

- 1 cup of broccoli has 27 calories and 8 grams of carbs (2 grams of fiber)
- 1 cup of pineapple has 80 calories and 21 grams of carbs (2 grams of fiber)
- 1 cup of golden potatoes has 110 calories and 26 grams of carbs (4 grams of fiber)
- 1 cup of cooked quinoa has 222 calories and 39 grams of carbs (5 grams of fiber)

Remember that the less active you are, the fewer starchy carbs and grains you'll likely need since they are more carbohydrate and calorie dense and generally have a higher glycemic load. The more active and insulin sensitive you are, the more carbs you can handle. This is why exercise is a vital part of health and liberates you to eat a much more varied diet with less risk of becoming overweight.

Now that I've covered the types of carbs I recommend reintroducing, let's discuss when to reintroduce carbohydrates after keto.

HOW DO YOU KNOW WHETHER YOU SHOULD STAY KETO?

Let me first emphasize that keto is not the only nutrition strategy for losing body fat and obtaining optimal health. Millions of people have successfully lost weight and gotten healthier while eating carbs.

In the last chapter, I discussed some reasons why you may want to consider bringing carbs back in. That being said, if you are on a ketogenic diet and have had improved health outcomes from it, here are a few reasons why you may want to stay keto longer:

- **You just plain feel amazing on keto.** How you feel matters. If you are doing keto, you're feeling the best you have in a long time, and your health is getting better and better, keep going. A lot of factors contribute to a person's nutritional needs, including many that are not yet fully understood, so there is value in simply doing what makes you feel amazing.

- **You have a medical reason to do keto.** If you are managing a disease, illness, or other health issue with a ketogenic diet, consult with a doctor or other health professional before making changes.

- **You still have a lot of weight to lose and keto is working.** Generally, the more obese you are, the less you can tolerate carbs without gaining weight. If you're in active fat-loss mode on keto, even if it's moving slowly, you might want to keep going until you've gotten closer to your goal weight and keto stops working.

Even if you start out feeling great on keto, or you currently do, there will likely come a time, somewhere along your keto journey, when that will change. You won't feel as good as you used to. Your results won't keep coming. And all of a sudden, you will wonder why this approach that used to make you feel so good isn't having that effect anymore.

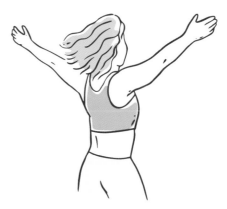

HOW MANY CARBS
SHOULD YOU EAT?

No one can confidently answer that question for you straight out of the gate. Our bodies are different, with different metabolic rates, hormonal environments, activity levels, stress levels, sleep quantity and quality, and more. All of these factors impact how many carbohydrates a person needs without spilling over into fat stores. So you'll have to play with it a little.

That being said, I generally tell people to start off by getting 20 percent of their total calories from carbohydrates (40 percent from fat, 40 percent from protein) and then increasing by 5 percent each week (subtracting 5 percent from fat) until they find a range that feels optimal. The four-week meal plan in this book does this each week, so you can figure it out for yourself. You might even consider doing each week of the meal plan for an entire month to really see how you feel on that particular ratio of fat and carbs.

HOW MANY CALORIES
DO YOU NEED?

Here is a baseline on how to calculate your total calories. You must play with these numbers to determine your body's unique threshold. I recommend slower fat loss with slight calorie deficits rather than extreme deficits that can lead to bingeing.

- **For fat loss:** Multiply your body weight in pounds × 10 to 12
- **For weight maintenance:** Multiply your body weight in pounds × 13 to 15
- **For mass/muscle gain:** Multiply your body weight in pounds × 16 to 18

The more muscle mass you have and the more active you are, the more likely it is that you will do better at the higher end of those ranges; those who are less active and less muscular should stick to the lower end.

THE GAME PLAN:
HOW TO FIND YOUR SWEET SPOT ON CARBS AFTER KETO

First, note the following:

- Your total calories will remain the same for all four weeks. Use the formulas just outlined to find the right starting number for you.

- You may add unlimited nonstarchy vegetables each week without tracking them if they do not cause bloating and gas. Depending on your gut microbial diversity, you may do extremely well with this approach, or you may get really bloated and have digestive issues by adding in too much fiber at once. If it's the latter, cut back.

- Prioritize carbohydrates from starchy vegetables, fruit, and whole grains. These foods will give you better results.

- Try to eat the same selection of carbohydrate sources throughout this experiment so you don't get thrown off if your body happens to prefer one carbohydrate source over another.

- Ideally, you should add the largest portion of carbs post-workout and combine them with protein. Eating carbs and protein within sixty minutes of your workout is ideal.

- If you're not very active and you don't have much muscle mass, you may not need as many carbs. Therefore, it's important to feel it out and experiment a little to find the amount that's best for you.

- As you go through the process, note how you are feeling. Did you feel better with lower carbs or higher carbs? How were your mood, sleep, exercise performance, energy, and digestion? Continue to experiment with your carb and fat levels and see which ratio makes you feel the best. This can also change during different periods of your life depending on stress, sleep habits, body composition, activity level, age, disease/illness, and other factors, so don't get pigeonholed into anything as your only approach for the rest of your life.

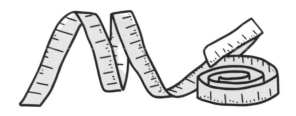

You will start with carbs at 20 percent of your total calories the first week—not much higher than keto—to avoid a drastic macronutrient shift, which can be hard on your gut. Each week, you will increase carbs by 5 percent while lowering fat by 5 percent. Protein will remain the same—40 percent of your calories—for the duration of the four weeks. This will allow you to stay full, build healthy neurotransmitters, recover from workouts, and build muscle without gaining body fat.

WEEK 1 MACROS:

- Protein: 40%
- Fat: 40%
- Carbs: 20%

WEEK 2 MACROS:

- Protein: 40%
- Fat: 35%
- Carbs: 25%

WEEK 3 MACROS:

- Protein: 40%
- Fat: 30%
- Carbs: 30%

WEEK 4 MACROS:

- Protein: 40%
- Fat: 25%
- Carbs: 35%

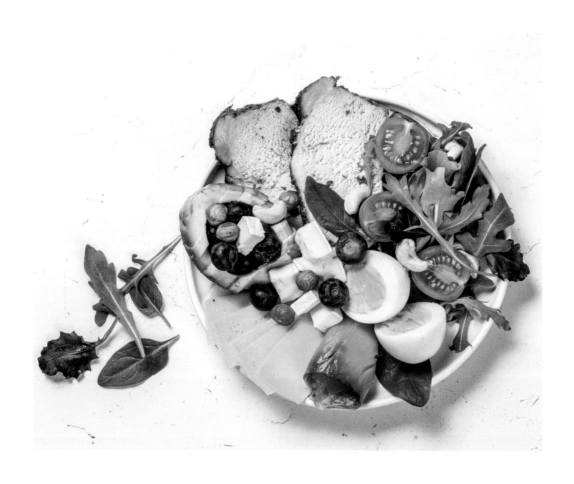

3: HOW TO BRING CARBS BACK IN AND
MATCH YOUR WORKOUTS WITH YOUR NUTRITION

Here are two examples:

	200-POUND PERSON SEEKING FAT LOSS WHO WANTS TO REINTRODUCE CARBS		150-POUND PERSON SEEKING FAT LOSS WHO WANTS TO REINTRODUCE CARBS	
WEEK 1	Calories:	2,000	Calories:	1,500
	Protein (40%):	200g	Protein (40%):	150g
	Fat (40%):	89g	Fat (40%):	67g
	Carbs (20%):	100g	Carbs (20%):	75g
WEEK 2	Calories:	2,000	Calories:	1,500
	Protein (40%):	200g	Protein (40%):	150g
	Fat (35%):	78g	Fat (35%):	58g
	Carbs (25%):	125g	Carbs (25%):	94g
WEEK 3	Calories:	2,000	Calories:	1,500
	Protein (40%):	200g	Protein (40%):	150g
	Fat (30%):	67g	Fat (30%):	50g
	Carbs (30%):	150g	Carbs (30%):	113g
WEEK 4	Calories:	2,000	Calories:	1,500
	Protein (40%):	200g	Protein (40%):	150g
	Fat (25%):	56g	Fat (25%):	42g
	Carbs (35%):	175g	Carbs (35%):	131g

MAXIMIZING ATHLETIC PERFORMANCE

If you are an athlete, and especially if you do high-intensity sports or exercise, eating carbohydrates in order to store more glycogen in your muscles is a smart move.

During intense intermittent exercise and throughout prolonged physical activity, muscle glycogen is broken down, causing glucose molecules to be released. Muscle cells then oxidize those glucose molecules to produce adenosine triphosphate (ATP), which is required for muscle contractions.

Athletes generally require more carbohydrates than the general population for maximum performance and recovery. You'll also want to consider the duration and intensity of the exercise you do when choosing carbohydrate amounts, and remember that you need fewer carbohydrates on rest days than on training days. For most athletes, I recommend exploring 150 grams of carbs per day and above. Increase that number by 25 grams one week at a time to find your sweet spot.

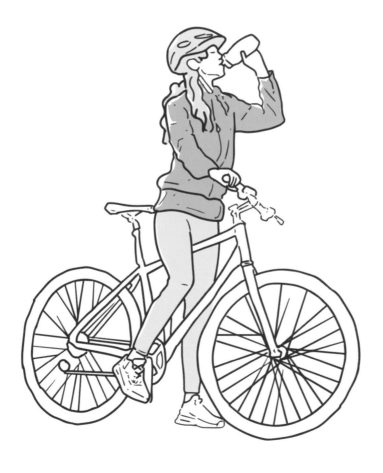

WHAT TO WATCH FOR AS
YOU BRING CARBS BACK IN

When you are reintroducing a food group that you have previously restricted, there will likely be some mental and physical reactions that you will want to be prepared for. Let's discuss.

CARBPHOBIA

I'm serious. This is a matter of the heart that I have seen over and over as a ketogenic diet specialist who helps people transition back into carbs after a keto phase. Many people are fearful of what will happen to them if they eat carbs again.

Sometimes people tell me that when they eat any carbs at all, they crave carbs like crazy. While, yes, technically, there can be biological reasons for this spike in cravings, particularly blood sugar, there is also another possibility. And that is because you have mentally restricted carbohydrates for so long, and you have missed all of your favorite foods (let's face it, pizza and bread taste really good). So, once that door is cracked, the floodgates break wide open. That is normal and can happen after a period of food restriction. It's important to give yourself permission to eat carbohydrates again without guilt or fear.

Also, if this happens to you during this period of reintroduction, ask yourself honestly whether you really feel worse with carbs—like vegetables, fruit, and potatoes—or if you feel worse every time you eat carbs because you end up going off the rails and eating a bunch of less healthy carbs, and way too many?

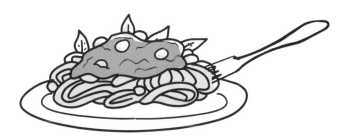

There are a lot of people out there who have developed disordered eating patterns from keto but aren't talking about it. So, if that's you—if you keep bingeing on all the things every single time you have a carb—I want you to consider whether keto is really improving your health, especially your mental health, your relationship with food, and your relationship with yourself.

Above all, having a healthy relationship with food, without fears around it or guilting or shaming yourself when you eat something that isn't "perfect," is a key to your overall health.

And if any fears around carbs creep back into your mind, remember that the healthiest populations in the world basically live on carbs—healthy carbs.

SLIGHT WEIGHT GAIN

As mentioned earlier, you will retain a little more water when you're eating carbs. Carbs pull water into your muscles—2 to 3 grams of water for every gram of carbohydrate stored in the body as glycogen. Don't freak out if you see the scale go up a few pounds when you reintroduce carbs. This is normal. Please do not be so obsessive about minor fluctuations in your weight that you pigeonhole yourself into a single dietary approach. The plus side is that you don't have to worry so much about getting dehydrated as you do on keto.

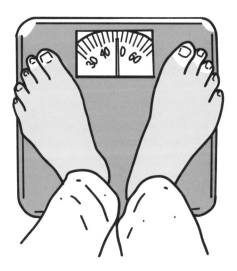

BLOATING OR DIGESTIVE CHANGES

Some bloating or digestive changes are to be expected. You are changing your macronutrient ratios just as you did when you switched to keto. Your body needs time to produce adequate amounts of amylase, the enzyme that helps break down carbs. Also, if you're really enjoying unlimited vegetables, bloating is almost certain to happen since your body isn't used to so much fiber. Your digestion should normalize in the first couple of weeks. If it doesn't, try cutting back on the veggies that make you bloat and switch to 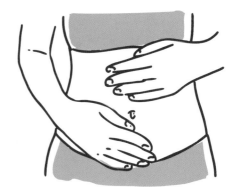 ones that don't. Remember that fiber in large quantities will make anyone bloat. You can take betaine hydrochloride and digestive enzymes, including amylase, to help with bloating during this transition.

As you build up your daily carbohydrate intake, I also recommend increasing the intensity of your workouts. More carbs will allow you to perform better at high-intensity interval training, weightlifting, sprinting, and other high-intensity sports.

I recommend pairing the four-week meal plan in Appendix C with the training plan that accompanies it to ensure your body actually has a need for those carbs. Using them in your workouts creates space in your muscles and liver for more carbs to come in, thus preventing body fat gain from eating carbs.

REFERENCES

1. David G. Le Couteur et al., "New Horizons: Dietary Protein, Ageing and the Okinawan Ratio," *Age and Ageing* 45, no. 4 (2016): 443–7, https://doi.org/10.1093/ageing/afw069.

2. Michael A. Conlon and Anthony R. Bird, "The Impact of Diet and Lifestyle on Gut Microbiota and Human Health," *Nutrients* 7, no. 1 (2014): 17–44, https://doi.org/10.3390/nu7010017.

3. Cecilie Kyrø et al., "Higher Whole-Grain Intake Is Associated with Lower Risk of Type 2 Diabetes Among Middle-Aged Men and Women: The Danish Diet, Cancer, and Health Cohort," *Journal of Nutrition* 148, no. 9 (2018): 1434–44, https://doi.org/10.1093/jn/nxy112.

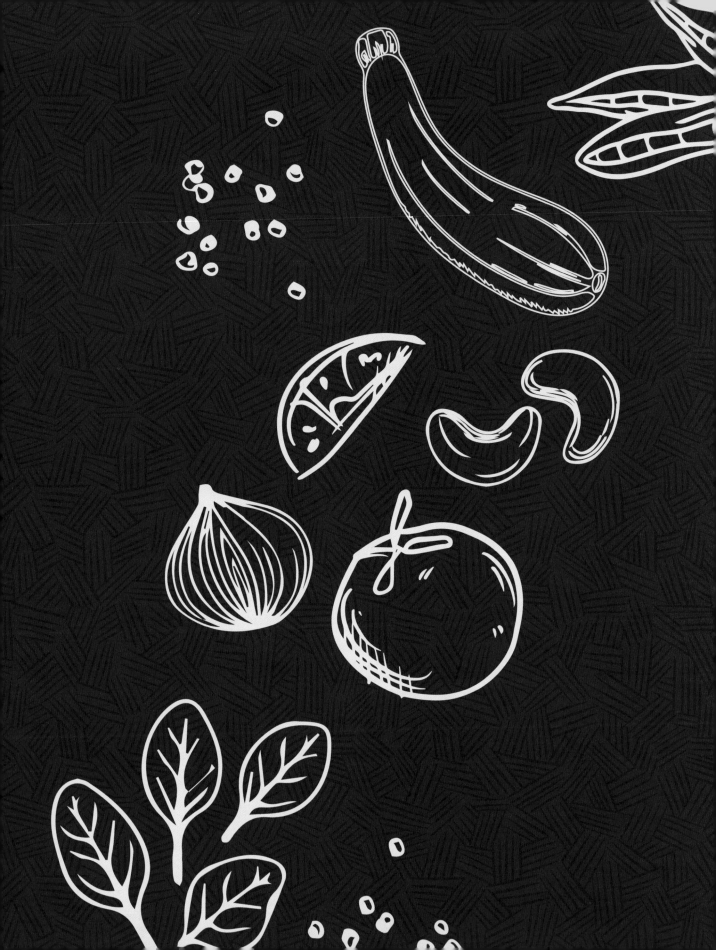

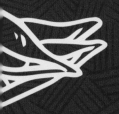

CHAPTER 4

WHERE TO GO FROM HERE: BRINGING BACK THE CARBS AND MAINTAINING METABOLIC FLEXIBILITY

After doing a keto phase and reintroducing carbohydrates in an optimal way through the four-week meal plan in this book, you may want to try some other dietary strategies to help you maintain metabolic flexibility. Metabolic flexibility is freedom. It is, in my opinion, the ultimate goal of our nutritional strategies. The goal is for our bodies to be able to run on carbs as their primary fuel source and feel amazing, and alternatively to be able to run on fat as their primary fuel source and feel just as wonderful. This is metabolic flexibility; this is how we free ourselves from feeling chronically dependent on consuming glucose for energy.

Our bodies were designed, masterfully, to transition into and out of ketosis. It keeps us insulin sensitive so that we can avoid diabetes and excess weight gain; it allows us to get used to eating according to physiological hunger, not "low blood sugar hunger," and experience all the benefits of both of those metabolic states, ketosis and glycolysis.

The process of transitioning between the two states should be effortless. So let me show you how to train your body to do it and gift yourself the freedom that comes with metabolic flexibility.

I've included a meal plan in this book to show you how to intelligently reintroduce the right kinds of carbohydrates after keto, gradually increasing carbs and decreasing fat each week over a period of four weeks. The gradual reintroduction gives your gut time to adjust to different macronutrient ratios so it can produce the right balance of enzymes to digest your food properly. It can take your body up to a couple of weeks to start producing more amylase, the enzyme in your saliva and excreted by your pancreas that helps you break down carbohydrates, to handle the new level of carbohydrates you're eating. So, if you slam your body with tons of carbohydrates all at once, you may not be able to break them down, which can lead to discomfort, gas, bloating, and constipation.

On top of this, if you suddenly and dramatically increase the amount of fiber you're consuming, you can almost certainly expect gas, bloating, and constipation. That will probably happen anyway, even with smaller increases in fiber, and it's normal; it's not necessarily a bad thing. Your body will slowly begin to increase the number of good bacteria that help you break down fiber. So don't be alarmed if you get some gas and bloating even as you increase carbohydrates and fiber gradually. Your body is simply adjusting.

Keep in mind that the types of carbohydrates you eat when reintroducing carbs will make or break the experience. It is imperative that you don't eat inflammatory carbohydrates, like processed foods and sugar, during this four-week reintroduction period. If you do, you will retain a ton of water, become inflamed, and feel like garbage. This, in my opinion, is why many people get "stuck" on keto. What starts out as a well-planned and well-timed sweet potato ends up with chips, ice cream, cookies, and candy being consumed with reckless abandon. And so these people jump to the conclusion that they feel terrible on carbs when really, they feel terrible on junk food.

As you increase carbohydrates, you'll also want to increase your exercise intensity to offset fat gain, continue to encourage insulin sensitivity, and use the insulin boost from the carbs to your advantage to build muscle.

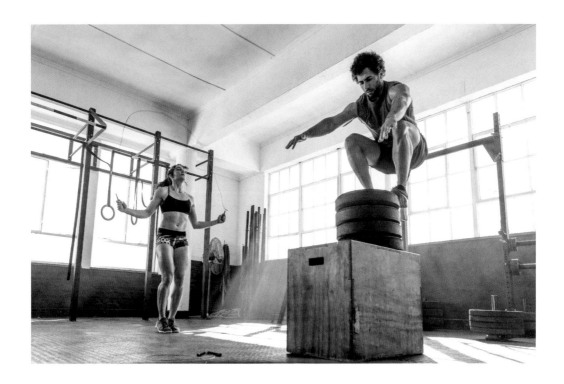

INSULIN IS YOUR FRIEND

Insulin is an energy-shuttling hormone. It often gets a bad rap, but it is an amazing energy delivery service for our cells. Our delivery guy takes glucose from our bloodstream and delivers it to the cells all over our bodies—our brains, other organs, and muscles—so they have energy to work correctly. About 20 percent of that glucose is used by our brains. Consuming about 120 grams of glucose, or about 480 calories' worth on a daily basis, the brain is the main user of glucose in the body. Our brains must have glucose for proper cognition, memory, and learning. When we create an environment inside of our bodies that makes our cells sensitive to insulin, this amazing hormone is definitely our friend!

When it comes to muscle growth, an insulin boost from eating carbs helps shuttle proteins into our muscles to begin muscle protein synthesis (muscle growth and repair). Carbs are also protein sparing, meaning the body looks to glycogen for energy instead of breaking down muscle for energy. Carbs also enhance exercise performance, which will help you hit the intensity levels in your weightlifting workouts required for muscle growth.

Once you have completed the four-week plan in this book, you may want to experiment to see if another approach might be your best groove for maintaining metabolic flexibility. Aside from plain ol' caloric restriction (which does work!), the following five approaches are my top recommended strategies for maintaining metabolic flexibility:

- Intermittent fasting
- One meal a day (OMAD)
- Targeted ketogenic diet (TKD)
- Cyclical ketogenic diet (CKD)
- Keto in and out: alternating between keto and a carbohydrate-based diet

I have included one-week meal plans and training plans for both the targeted ketogenic diet and the cyclical ketogenic diet so you can see what those look like when done optimally; see Appendixes A and B.

I have not included a meal plan for intermittent fasting or OMAD because you can do it with any nutritional and training approach. You can pair it with keto, low carb, moderate carb, or high carb. Play with it and see what feels best for you. Most people who intermittent fast as a lifestyle do it so they don't have to worry so much about macronutrient or calorie counting. The longer fasting window helps with insulin sensitivity; it also helps you avoid overconsuming calories. Bear in mind, however, that you can still consume too many calories even when intermittent fasting. Keeping track of your calories and macros in the beginning may help you get a feel for what works for you.

Experiment with any of these options for at least a month to see what is a great fit. In the following sections, I describe in detail why you might consider each one, the benefits and drawbacks, how to execute it, and how to work out to optimally match your nutritional approach.

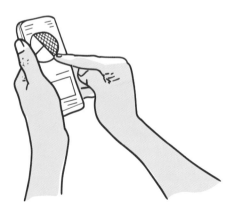

INTERMITTENT FASTING

Intermittent fasting is time-restricted eating. It means you eat only during a certain window of hours each day. Most people start out with a twelve-hour window, such as eating only between 8 a.m. and 8 p.m. After that, you can slowly shrink the window by one hour every few days until you get to an eight-hour window, such as eating only between 11 a.m. and 7 p.m. Sometimes people restrict their eating window even further, but an eight-hour window is a typical protocol for intermittent fasting.

Before I jump into the research, I will say that intermittent fasting has become a way of life for me, and I really enjoy it. I'm not militant about it, but I typically do not eat my first meal until somewhere around noon. I have coffee or a caffeinated pre-workout drink before heading to the gym. The combo of caffeine and exercise has a tremendous appetite-suppressing effect, making it almost effortless for me to intermittent fast. Then I wait until I get good and hungry to eat—somewhere between 11 a.m. and 1 p.m. And that is typically a large, satiating meal with lots of animal protein and vegetables, capped off with some berries and dark chocolate—often over Greek yogurt for more protein. I tend to eat again at around 4 p.m. and have another very similar large meal. I sometimes have small snacks in between, but I try to avoid that. I'm so satiated by my 4 p.m. meal that it keeps me full enough until bedtime. The lack of eating late at night is optimal for digestion and helps me get appropriately sleepy for bed; I think it is one of the keys to my having been able to maintain a lean physique for many years.

The other reasons I enjoy intermittent fasting are that I really like the feeling of getting nice and full from a meal versus eating smaller meals that leave me wanting more. The feast-or-famine approach ensures that I don't overeat without having to track anything, and it makes my life so much easier. I also love the energy levels and cognitive clarity that I experience when I eat this way. When I don't intermittent fast and just eat randomly throughout the day, my cognitive function and energy levels are just not as high.

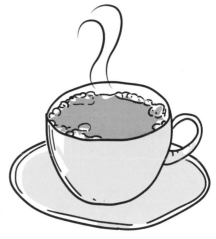

In a nutshell, intermittent fasting is a simple life strategy that keeps me lean and performing at high levels in my work life without having to stress over calorie and macro tracking all the time. It works for me.

THE RESEARCH BEHIND INTERMITTENT FASTING

There is a lot of buzz about intermittent fasting in the nutrition world right now. From celebrities to health coaches to your next-door neighbor's blog, it seems like everyone is talking about it. At the time of writing this book, a Google search for "intermittent fasting" produced over 12 million results. So let's dive into the research and see what all the buzz is about. There are a small number of negative results, but overall, the results are extremely favorable.

In terms of negatives, besides the study showing muscle loss that I mentioned earlier, a 2020 study of 116 overweight and obese men and women compared the results of time-restricted eating and consistent meal timing over the course of three months. The researchers found that the time-restricted eating group lost a small amount of weight—an average of 2 to 3.5 pounds—while the consistent meal-timing group did not. However, 65 percent of the weight lost came from lean mass, about double the normal amount of lean mass lost during a weight-reduction period. It's important to note, though, that other studies suggest this can be offset by eating enough protein during your eating window.[1] (Other studies of people who ate adequate protein while intermittent fasting showed no muscle loss at all.) These are the only "negative" research results I have been able to find on the topic.

As a side note, I have zero problems getting in 150 grams of protein or more during my eating window, which is within a good range for someone like me who weighs about 150 pounds, has a decent amount of muscle mass, and is physically active. I am a big advocate for protein, especially for active people, and even more for people who regularly weight train. Exercise increases the body's protein requirements, so if eating enough protein is hard for you, working out can boost your cravings for it. I emphasize the importance of protein because eating more protein has been an absolute game changer for me and my clients in terms of improved body composition, feeling better mentally and emotionally, and feeling fuller for longer on fewer calories. And the research agrees—getting enough protein is the key to successful body composition transformation while intermittent fasting.

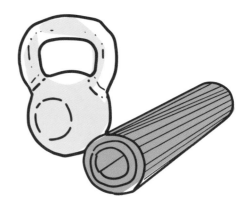

Now let's discuss the positive research results in regard to intermittent fasting, which came in spades. Check these out:

- A study put elite cyclists on an eight-hour eating window and found that it resulted in reduced body weight and fat mass percentage with no change in fat-free mass (in other words, no muscle loss). It's also significant that the performance of the intermittent fasters did not drop; they saw an improvement in peak power output:body weight ratio due to the weight loss. The study also tested for markers of immune health and found that the intermittent fasting group had a significant improvement in immune system biomarkers compared to the control group of elite cyclists who weren't intermittent fasting.[2]

- A 2014 review of the scientific literature found that intermittent fasting results in weight loss of 3 to 8 percent of the subjects over three to twenty-four weeks. That is a huge amount. It's also significant that the subjects lost 4 to 7 percent of their waist circumference, which indicates a loss of belly fat, the harmful fat that surrounds the organs and leads to disease. The review also showed that fasting blood sugar was reduced by 3 to 6 percent and fasting insulin was reduced by 20 to 31 percent. These changes are extremely beneficial for metabolic health and disease prevention.[3]

- A 2017 meta-analysis of thirty-five studies examined weight changes and changes in metabolic markers during Ramadan (a month during which Muslims engage in time-restricted eating, fasting from sunrise to sunset). This analysis found that intermittent fasting enhanced weight loss and reduced basal concentrations of many metabolic biomarkers associated with chronic disease, such as insulin and glucose.[4]

- A study on diabetic rats showed that intermittent fasting protected against kidney damage, one of the most serious complications of diabetes.[5]

- Several studies have shown that intermittent fasting may enhance the body's resistance to oxidative stress, aka inflammation, the driver of all sorts of disease.[6]

- Multiple studies have shown that intermittent fasting improves numerous cardiovascular health markers, including blood pressure, total and LDL cholesterol, triglycerides, inflammatory markers, and blood sugar levels.[7]

- Several studies have found that intermittent fasting and dietary restriction enhance brain function through the increase and growth of new nerve cells.[8]

- Studies of rodents have shown that intermittent fasting extends life span.[9]

- Finally, an in-depth review of the scientific literature on intermittent fasting published in the *New England Journal of Medicine* confirms that intermittent fasting improves metabolism, lowers blood sugar, lessens inflammation, clears out toxins and damaged cells, lowers diabetes and cancer risk, and enhances brain function.[10]

HOW TO APPROACH INTERMITTENT FASTING

As you go through your metabolic optimization journey, it's up to you whether to do intermittent fasting the entire time. You can do it while you're on a ketogenic diet, or you can eat normally. I recommend trying intermittent fasting and seeing what it does for you. It will be uncomfortable at first, but many people find it becomes a life groove that they never want to change.

I recommend making your eating window earlier in the day rather than later because we become increasingly less insulin sensitive as we approach nighttime sleep. Do what works for you, but I like to end my eating window by 5 p.m. Eating between 11 a.m. and 5 p.m. or even 12 p.m. and 4 p.m. is typical for me.

If you are in the keto phase of your journey, having a longer fasting window will help you dig further into ketosis. If you're not in your keto phase, depending on how many carbs you consume during your eating window and your activity level, you may drift into ketosis during your fasting window, which is amazing for metabolic health. The only way to know for sure is to check your ketone levels. For that, I recommend the Keto-Mojo meter or a similar device that you can use to check your blood sugar and ketone levels any time you want by means of a finger prick.

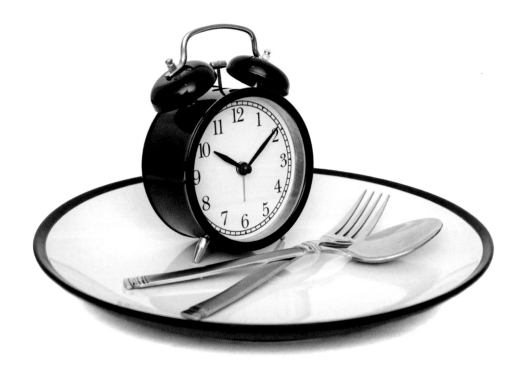

Here's what a typical day of intermittent fasting looks like for me:

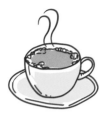

5 a.m.—I have a small black coffee while I do my morning routine (meditation, gratitude, personal development, and goal setting/planning).

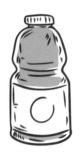

7 a.m.—Gym time with a pre-workout drink. (Yes, it is caffeinated. I am a fast metabolizer of caffeine, and I have been doing this for years without noticing any negative consequences. Caffeine is a fat mobilizer and is clinically proven to enhance athletic performance, which is why I make it a part of my routine. I make sure to stay on top of my minerals so I don't develop adrenal issues. I take the Upgraded Formulas Hair Mineral Test yearly to make sure I'm within the normal range. And because I know I'm going to be asked, I use Honey Badger stevia-sweetened pre-workout. [See Appendix D for discount codes for both products if you're interested.])

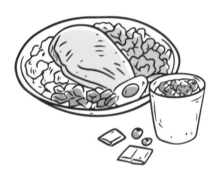

11 a.m. to 12 p.m.—I typically have my first meal of the day around this time. It is usually a big stir-fry with lots of vegetables and lean protein cooked in a quality cooking fat like avocado oil, olive oil, or ghee and topped with a little guacamole for extra fat. I sometimes include carbs, like sweet potatoes or rice. I go intuitively on this. If I'm really craving carbs, I go for it; if not, I pass. I usually have protein-rich yogurt with berries in this meal also—along with some sort of fat-filled small dessert like dark chocolate or a couple of tablespoons of nut butter.

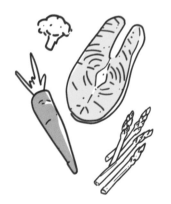

4 p.m.—I repeat the same meal as before, swapping out different proteins and plants for nutrient variety.

That's it! In the evenings I usually drink a huge cup of water with my minerals from Upgraded Formulas, trace mineral drops, and an electrolyte powder, and sometimes sip on tea. This helps keep me satiated and helps me routinely get in my minerals and electrolytes, and I wake up the next day feeling amazing.

My eating window is pretty small, usually four to seven hours, but I have been intermittent fasting for years, so baby-step it if you are new to fasting. I also don't force myself to intermittent fast. If I wake up incredibly hungry on certain days, I go ahead and eat. And of course, sometimes I eat later in the evening, but that's rare. I never feel as good when I do that, so I don't do it often or recommend it to others. There isn't one right way to intermittent fast. I recommend trying it along your journey and seeing what works for you.

Even if you decide intermittent fasting isn't your thing, I really do recommend not getting into the habit of waiting until super late in the day to eat. In my experience, it is difficult to make good food choices when your willpower is low. As I mentioned previously, you are also less sensitive to insulin at night, so more of your food is likely to go toward fat storage than it would if you ate earlier in the day and ended your eating window earlier. I have found that stopping eating earlier in the day really helps people stay lean, and it helps set your circadian rhythm so you can fall asleep sooner. But again, play with it and see what works for *you.*

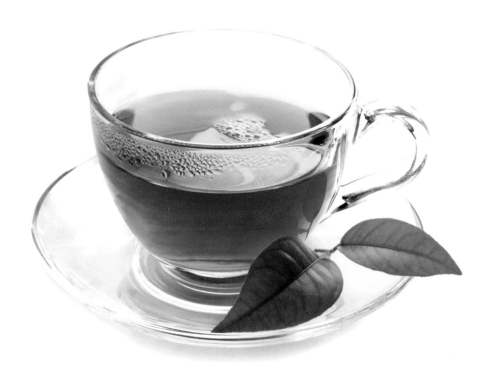

ONE MEAL A DAY
(OMAD)

One meal a day (OMAD) is just what it sounds like—you eat only once per day. This isn't an approach I recommend doing long term, but it can be a useful temporary tool for training your body to transition into ketosis without having to do a full-on ketogenic diet phase. It also helps with impulse control.

OMAD is extremely simple and easy to follow, training your body to transition into ketosis effectively and giving you some of the benefits of time-restricted eating. The reason I don't recommend doing OMAD long term is that research has shown some negative outcomes, such as increased blood pressure, increased total and LDL cholesterol, and elevated morning glucose levels.[11] I also don't recommend doing OMAD if you have a history of disordered eating, as it may trigger a binge-and-restrict cycle to unhealthy levels.

Overall, eating two or three meals throughout the day has been shown to be more beneficial for human health than one meal,[12] but a short phase of OMAD, such as one to three weeks at a time, may be a smart strategy for maintaining metabolic flexibility and training your body on what to do in the absence of a constant food supply.

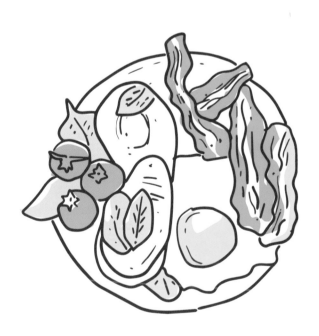

Now, if you are going to try OMAD, remember there aren't any "rules" here; you can make it look however you want. Some people classify a four-hour eating window as OMAD, some do a two-hour eating window, and some put it all into only one meal. It doesn't really matter. The idea is that you have a short feasting period and the rest of the day, you just let your body use it up—along with some stored body fat.

I did OMAD for several months during the COVID-19 lockdown when all of the gyms were closed. My exercise output went down drastically because of the closures, and along with it went my appetite. I naturally fell into an OMAD pattern since I already intermittent fasted, so I just rolled with it. I actually lost 15 pounds in six weeks! I was pretty astonished. It was the lowest my weight has been in years. My exercise output during that time included lots of walking around the lake by my house, an occasional run, and a few bodyweight HIIT workouts, but it was considerably lower than normal. I did not lift any weights because I didn't have any at home.

I did not track my body composition during this time, and I'm sure some of the weight I lost was muscle mass loss due to the lack of resistance training, but I could tell by the way I looked that I was losing body fat, too. I was very lean. I also noticed that my energy was up, my drive and motivation were up, and my mood was enhanced. I honestly started falling in love with this approach. I literally ate whatever I wanted during my feasting window with zero guilt.

I did make sure that I packed in a *ton* of protein during that feast, and I was mindful of eating vegetables and fruits for phytonutrients. I admit, though, that sometimes I would eat my old favorites, like pizza or cookies—and I still lost 15 pounds! I also made sure I was on top of my supplement game so my body was getting the vitamins and minerals it needed, especially on those pizza days.

After a while, though, I noticed that calories did still matter. Sometimes I would extend my eating window to four hours, sometimes I did two, and sometimes I did one. I definitely noticed quick changes in my body in terms of fat loss when I kept to a one-hour eating window. On the days I ate within a two- to four-hour window, I found I could still really take some calories down, and my weight would stall or even go up during those periods.

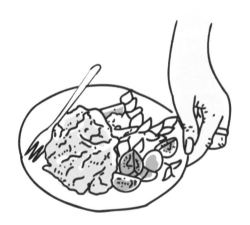

4: **WHERE TO GO FROM HERE:** BRINGING BACK THE CARBS AND MAINTAINING METABOLIC FLEXIBILITY

I honestly felt so good using this approach that I almost wrote an e-book about it. It's simple. It's efficient. It takes no planning. It's extremely effective for fat loss. And it has a long list of health benefits, as described in the intermittent fasting section.

There was only one reason I didn't: I experienced a disruption in my menstrual cycle while doing OMAD, which had never happened to me before. I am very regular, like clockwork. But during my OMAD experience, I started spotting irregularly, and my cycle started two weeks after my previous period. That change concerned me. Even when I later did a bodybuilding bikini competition and combined extreme calorie deficits with heavy exercise, my cycle didn't change at all. I was on my period while I was onstage at 10 percent body fat! So, although I don't know for sure why my cycle was disrupted during my OMAD experiment, it made me apprehensive about recommending the approach on a broad scale, especially to women.

So I am sharing this experience as food for thought if you decide to try OMAD. I will put it this way: there are no trophies here. If it's not working for you, don't worry about it. Go back to a normal eating schedule.

I will also add that if you're the type of person who can't ever finish a meal and you pick at your food like a bird, OMAD probably isn't a smart strategy for you. We want to be mindful of nutritional deficiencies. I'm the kind of person who can seriously take down some food, and I already love the feast-or-famine approach to nutrition, so eating a lot within a small window was no problem for me. I also have a very efficient gut with great motility, so consider that for yourself as well. If you have digestive issues, this probably isn't a good strategy for you. The meal you eat is generally a pretty hefty feast since all of your nutrients have to come in that meal.

Remember too that food quality is paramount. Supplementation is wise as well so you cover your micronutrient bases. I recommend taking a quality multivitamin and fish or krill oil as a minimum supplement protocol.

Most people on OMAD generally eat this meal within an hour, but some broaden the mealtime to up to several hours. If you're reading this and thinking, "That sounds absolutely horrible," honestly, it's probably not for you. No worries, though; there are plenty of other approaches for maintaining metabolic flexibility. That said, there are many people out there who tend to do OMAD naturally or are very attracted to the idea. If that's you, OMAD may be a tool in your metabolically flexible toolkit that you use from time to time as a reset.

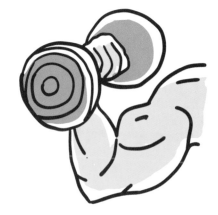

It's up to you whether to track calories or macros or not on OMAD. However, *not* having to track calories or macros while still allowing your body to run on fat for fuel is what attracts people to this approach. No matter what you eat, you will likely drift into ketosis at some point since you are fasting for twenty to twenty-three hours each day.

If you feel OMAD is too stressful on your body, please choose another approach.

TARGETED KETOGENIC DIET (TKD)

This is a very popular approach for the athletic keto crowd. The idea behind the targeted ketogenic diet (TKD) is to enhance athletic performance and recovery by adding a little more carbohydrate than the traditional ketogenic diet only in the peri-workout window (before or after your workout) while eating keto the rest of the time. I recommend getting fully keto-adapted for at least four weeks before beginning this approach.

The amount of carbs to eat around the workout depends on the individual. The amount of muscle mass you have, your basal metabolic rate, and the level of exercise intensity and volume you perform are all factors. Generally, most ketogenic athletes consume 25 to 50 grams of carbohydrates within an hour before or after exercise for this approach. Please remember that exercise intensity *matters*—if you are going really intense in the gym, doing a workout with a very high heart rate, it will probably warrant a higher carb intake pre- or post-workout. If you had a light workout, you won't need as many carbs, if any. You have to play with the amounts to see what feels and works best for you.

WHEN TO EAT THOSE EXTRA CARBS

There seems to be a lot of confusion about *when* to eat these extra carbohydrates for optimal performance, and that is understandable because there are different ways to look at it. I'll share the bases for post-workout carbs and pre-workout carbs so you can be educated about how they both work in the body, and possibly try both methods to see which works better for you.

Here is some evidence for eating carbohydrates in the hour *following* your workout:
A 2014 study measuring the performance of cyclists based on pre- or post-workout carbohydrate consumption found that when the athletes consumed carbohydrates one hour before exercise, there was a larger drop in their blood sugar, which led to impaired performance. When they ate carbohydrates post-workout, within one hour of exercise, there was a significant increase in muscle glycogen replenishment and a decrease in muscle recovery time. When the athletes waited more than an hour to replenish with carbs, however, they experienced longer muscle recovery times.[13]

Post-workout carbs spike insulin, which supports muscle protein synthesis when your body needs it most. Carbohydrates also blunt the rise of cortisol, which is a catabolic or "breaking down" hormone, meaning it can break down muscle tissue. This is not what you want. By hindering cortisol production with carbohydrates, not only do you allow your body to repair and grow muscle tissue more successfully, but you also help protect it against negative consequences of elevated cortisol. Those consequences include impaired cognitive function, disrupted sleep, lower immune function, increased abdominal fat, and worsening blood sugar imbalances. This is particularly important given that studies have shown cortisol levels increase more on a ketogenic diet in response to exercise than on a standard diet that includes carbohydrates.[14]

The post-workout carbs approach is my preferred method of TKD for these reasons. The magic of muscle growth doesn't happen in your workout; it happens in the recovery period. Eating carbohydrates after your workout not only helps you enhance that recovery and stimulate muscle protein synthesis, but also gets stored muscle glycogen ready to be used as fuel for tomorrow's workout.

Now, because I like to give you as many options to consider as possible, I will share that some athletes prefer to use fast-acting, readily available simple carbohydrates, such as dextrose or glucose, immediately before and during intense training for a few reasons.

The theory behind that preference is that you want to provide your body with immediate glucose in the bloodstream to fuel performance instead of forcing it to mobilize adrenaline in order to release stored muscle glycogen into the bloodstream to be used for athletic performance. This circles back to our earlier conversation about cortisol. The reason for avoiding extra catecholamine release for the purpose of releasing stored glycogen into the bloodstream is that when catecholamines are released, the body also releases cortisol, which is catabolic. Some proponents of this idea want to *prevent* a large rise of cortisol with carbs in order to put themselves in an anabolic state.

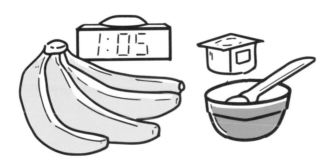

I *want* my body to release catecholamines (adrenaline) during exercise for the performance boost, and I prefer to stimulate muscle protein synthesis and blunt post-workout cortisol production by consuming carbs and protein *after* my workout. But if this pre-workout carbohydrate idea appeals to you (and I recommend you try both so you can see which one works better for you), eating "fast" carbs like dextrose and glucose are key; you don't want complex carbohydrates in this scenario. You want an instant source of glucose in your bloodstream that your muscles can easily utilize for the workout. You'll also want to favor glucose over fructose, as fructose fills up liver glycogen, and you want to provide glucose to your *muscles* more than your liver. This will not only boost your exercise performance but also allow you to get back into ketosis more quickly when the workout has ended since liver glycogen is what prevents the production of ketones.

BUILDING MUSCLE USING A TARGETED KETO APPROACH

Whether you choose pre- or post-workout carbohydrates as part of your targeted ketogenic diet, a key benefit of adding in carbs is creating an insulin response, which activates a protein called mTOR. mTOR induces muscle protein synthesis and puts the body in an anabolic, or muscle-building, state instead of a catabolic, or muscle-wasting, state. Many people are afraid of going out of ketosis. However, if you are not using keto therapeutically, this isn't something to fear. In fact, it can enhance your sports performance, recovery, and body composition.

If you try the pre-workout carb approach, I recommend consuming 10 to 50 grams of an easily digestible simple carbohydrate immediately before your workout. Continuing to sip on it during your workout is okay, too. The best quick-carb options for fueling muscle glycogen without filling liver glycogen are dextrose, glucose (which is dextrose bound to water), maltodextrin, and potato starch.

I recommend picking up a supplement such as highly branched cyclic dextrin and adding it to your pre-workout drink when doing this approach. Highly branched cyclic dextrin is an advanced type of maltodextrin that is digested very quickly and sends a steady stream of fuel to your muscles. It requires very little water for digestion, which means more water stays where your body needs it during exercise—in your muscles, not in your large intestine.

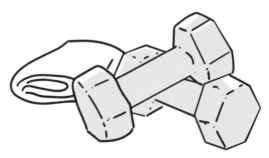

4: WHERE TO GO FROM HERE: BRINGING BACK THE CARBS AND MAINTAINING METABOLIC FLEXIBILITY

While I'm on the topic of keto and athletic performance, I want to remind you that you may not need carbohydrates at all to perform well and build muscle on keto. Research has shown that protein, especially the amino acid leucine, can spike insulin just like carbohydrates do.[15] Many ketogenic athletes simply supplement with leucine before, during, or after their training sessions. The only difference with leucine is that if you're aiming to refill muscle glycogen after your workout to fuel tomorrow's performance (the post-workout-carbs approach), you won't be getting that glycogen refill.

In regard to glycogen and athletic performance, a study that Dr. Jeff Volek published in a 2016 issue of the journal *Metabolism* is noteworthy. The study revealed that ten ultra-endurance athletes who had been following a ketogenic diet for at least six months had muscle glycogen levels at rest that were similar to the control group's. The study also found that glycogen levels *recovered* at the same rate in the keto group as they did in the control group, despite the fact that the keto group consumed a diet containing 5 percent carbohydrates while the control group ate a diet containing 50 percent carbohydrates.[16] That's pretty astonishing! The athletes showed a higher fat oxidation rate and a lower carbohydrate oxidation rate during exercise. The researchers concluded that endurance athletes could maintain normal muscle glycogen content, utilization, and recovery after a longer adaptation to a ketogenic diet. Food for thought! Especially for endurance athletes.

But what about ketogenic athletes who perform at high intensities, such as those who do high-volume weightlifting, CrossFit, sprinting, and high-intensity interval training, which rely heavily on anaerobic metabolism? Supplementing with carbohydrates may be a smart idea for them because ketones and fat cannot be metabolized anaerobically. Keep in mind, however, that some people do not experience performance decreases on keto, even in high-power-output sports. Some report *increases* in strength and athletic performance after transitioning to a ketogenic diet. It is hypothesized that this may be due to a systemic reduction in inflammation in those individuals.

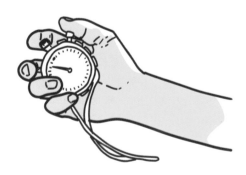

Research has also shown that it is possible to build muscle on a standard ketogenic diet. In one study, a ketogenic diet was compared to a traditional Western diet during a ten-week resistance training period in healthy young males.[17] After ten weeks, the ketogenic group gained 2.4 percent lean body mass and reduced their fat mass by 2.2 kilograms, similar to the group eating a Western diet. Strength and power also increased to the same extent in the ketogenic diet and Western diet groups.

I'm sharing these findings and possible solutions with you so you'll know you have options. Different bodies respond a bit differently to various nutritional approaches, so I want to give you as many choices as possible to find long-term solutions that feel optimal for you. A targeted ketogenic diet is enjoyable for many people who love the anti-inflammatory aspect of keto while still supporting athletic performance with carbohydrates. And please remember, temporarily going out of ketosis is not a bad thing. The entire point of metabolic flexibility is to be able to run on carbs like a boss *and* run on fat like a boss, utilizing the full capacity of your metabolism.

Like all dietary approaches, I encourage you to do some self-experimentation and see what works best for you.

In Appendix A, you'll find a One-Week Targeted Ketogenic Diet Meal Plan that shows you what a well-formulated targeted ketogenic diet looks like. I've also included a One-Week Targeted Ketogenic Diet Training Plan so you can see how to boost exercise intensity with the added carbohydrates.

The training plan is geared toward intermediate to advanced gym-goers, with five training sessions throughout the week. If this is too much for you, feel free to choose two to three training sessions to begin with and work your way up. Getting so sore that you can barely operate is not optimal. You want to feel the stimulus, but not so much that you can't perform in your next workout. Remember, on the days you don't do any high-intensity exercise, you don't need extra carbs, so follow a normal ketogenic diet on those days. (The plan is set for these days to be Tuesday and Thursday.)

The meal plan utilizes a post-workout-carbs targeted keto approach. Since most people work out in the morning, breakfast is the higher-carbohydrate post-workout meal. Feel free to switch it around if you work out later in the day. Consume your higher-carbohydrate meal within one hour of your workout.

I've included examples for both a 1,500-calorie and a 2,000-calorie diet. Adjust them as necessary to fit your caloric needs.

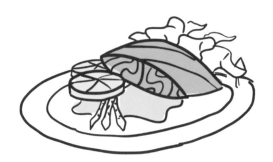

Your Targeted Ketogenic Diet Training Plan Schedule

Monday: Lower Body Weight Training

Tuesday: Walking Recovery Day (regular keto, no added carbs today)

Wednesday: High-Intensity Interval Training: Functional Circuit

Thursday: Walking Recovery Day (regular keto, no added carbs today)

Friday: Upper Body Weight Training

Saturday: High-Intensity Interval Training: Cardio

Sunday: Total Body Weight Training

Your Targeted Ketogenic Diet Meal Plan Guidelines

How to configure your calories:

- **For fat loss:** Multiply your body weight in pounds by 10. If you are not losing fat on this number of calories, or if the restriction is way too intense and you're absolutely starving, play with your calorie intake a little, moving it up or down until you find your sweet spot.

- **For weight maintenance:** Multiply your body weight in pounds by 13 or 14. You may have to move your calorie intake up or down a little until you find your sweet spot.

- **For mass gain:** Multiply your body weight in pounds by 15 or 16. You may have to move your calorie intake up or down a little until you find your sweet spot.

How to set your macros:

ON THE DAYS YOU WORK OUT:

- 55% fat
- 30% protein
- 15% carbs (mostly in your post-workout window)

ON THE DAYS YOU DON'T WORK OUT/WALKING ONLY:

- 65% fat
- 30% protein
- 5% carbs

You can choose your own foods or use the meal plan I've provided to get started on a post-workout carbohydrate targeted ketogenic diet.

Please see Appendix A for your One-Week Targeted Ketogenic Diet Meal Plan and Training Plan.

CYCLICAL KETOGENIC DIET (CKD)

A cyclical ketogenic diet means that you eat keto most days, but once or twice a week, you eat high-carb and low-fat. You eat the same number of calories you usually do, just swapping carbs for fat.

The high-carb days are often referred to as "carb-ups." The types of carbs you eat on those days will make or break this approach. If you eat a bunch of low-quality, inflammatory, processed carbs, you will feel like crap. High-quality, nutrient-dense carbohydrates, on the other hand, should make you feel amazing.

Some people do a high-carb day once a week; others opt for twice a week. You can try both options to see which setup feels better to you. Typically, the harder you work out and the leaner you are, the more you will benefit from more frequent carb-ups.

Remember that it's not a free-for-all; you won't just eat your normal high-fat diet and add carbs on top of it. The high-carb days will definitely feel different. You'll be eating very little fat on those days. This is key for avoiding calorie excess and accumulating body fat from this approach. So please be mindful.

The purpose of the cyclical ketogenic diet is to use carbs as a tool to maximize muscle growth and athletic performance while getting the benefits of the standard ketogenic diet. It's also a great way to maintain metabolic flexibility through diet variation. It can be an awesome approach for people who love keto but want to have some carbs sometimes, too.

Here's how you do it:

- Monday–Thursday: Keto
- Friday–Saturday: High-carb, low-fat
- Sunday: Fast to get back into ketosis

One important caveat is that the cyclical ketogenic diet needs to be paired with exercise! If you're not going to be training on Friday and Saturday, this approach is not for you; just stick with regular keto. However, if you're an active person who works out, cyclical keto can be an incredible approach.

Here's what you need to know about types of carbohydrates and carbohydrate timing:

On Friday, you want to include some high-glycemic carbs to replenish your glycogen stores. In the second twenty-four hours of eating carbohydrates, however, stick with low-glycemic, complex carbs to avoid fat gain, keep your insulin levels stable, and hold less water under your skin.[18]

As for timing, you can eat your carbohydrates as you please throughout the day. However, make sure that your first carb-up begins immediately following training. A delay of even two hours causes glycogen resynthesis to be 45 percent slower.[19]

In regard to training, you should do a total body workout on both Friday and Saturday. Your Friday workout should be performed before your first carb-up; your Saturday workout can be at any time during the day. Make sure you eat a carbohydrate-rich meal and pair it with protein, ideally within sixty minutes after the training session has ended.

In Appendix B, I've included a One-Week Cyclical Ketogenic Diet Meal Plan and Training Plan to show you what a well-formulated cyclical keto diet and training schedule looks like. Remember that prioritizing whole foods is the game changer here. You will get better body composition results and feel better mentally when you prioritize real foods.

I've included examples for both a 1,500-calorie and a 2,000-calorie diet. Adjust them as necessary to fit your caloric needs.

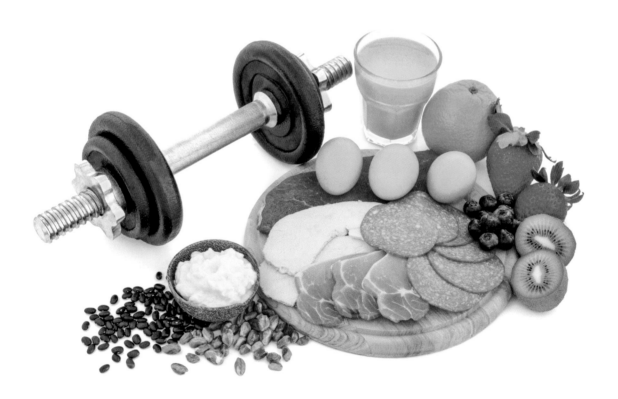

Your Cyclical Ketogenic Diet Training Plan Schedule

Monday: Keto-Specific Lower Body Training

Tuesday: Walking Recovery Day

Wednesday: Keto-Specific Upper Body Training

Thursday: Walking Recovery Day

Friday: Total Body Training*

Saturday: Total Body Training*

Sunday: Rest

These workouts are mandatory or you don't get your high-carb day. Do your Friday workout before your first carb-up. Your Saturday workout may be done at any time.

Your Cyclical Ketogenic Diet Meal Plan Guidelines

How to configure your calories:

- For fat loss: Multiply your body weight in pounds by 10. If you are not losing fat on this number of calories, or the restriction is way too intense and you're absolutely starving, play with your calorie intake a little, moving it up or down until you find your sweet spot.

- For weight maintenance: Multiply your body weight in pounds by 13 or 14. You may have to move your calorie intake up or down a little until you find your sweet spot.

- For mass gain: Multiply your body weight in pounds by 15 or 16. You may have to move your calorie intake up or down a little until you find your sweet spot.

How to set your macros:

- Monday–Thursday: Keto—65% fat, 30% protein, 5% carbs
- Friday: High-carb—65% carbs, 20% protein, 15% fat
- Saturday: High-carb—50% carbs, 30% protein, 20% fat
- Sunday: Fast to get back into ketosis. You can either fast the entire day or break your fast at dinner with a ketogenic meal.

Please see Appendix B for your One-Week Cyclical Ketogenic Diet Meal Plan and Training Plan.

KETO IN AND OUT: PERIODICALLY ALTERNATING BETWEEN KETO AND A BALANCED DIET

Keto in and out is another approach that I recommend trying after you have fully adapted to ketosis and feel you are no longer getting results from keto. It is for those who really want to maintain metabolic flexibility.

The length of time someone might do keto is highly individual. The more body fat you have and the higher your fasting blood sugar is, the longer you will likely benefit from the ketogenic approach. The minimum amount of time I recommend doing keto is one month. If, after completing that first month, you have excellent fasting glucose (under 90 mg/dL), are not experiencing improvements in body composition, and don't feel as optimal on keto, you will want to experiment with this approach and reintroduce carbohydrates, just like I show you how to do in the four-week meal plan in this book.

The meal plan in Appendix C outlines how to do so with the right kinds of carbs. Showing you how to eat in a healthy way that gets results after keto is the main purpose of this book! I want you to see how to bring carbohydrates back into your life in an optimal way. So many people go off the rails with processed carbs after keto because they have been restricted for so long. I see way too many people get pigeonholed into keto because they feel lost and aimless once they start reintroducing carbohydrates. All of a sudden, all the carbs they had been eliminating are back on the table, and soon they find themselves eating pizza and donuts, gaining weight, and turning back to keto. This all-or-nothing approach ruins everything! You may find it helpful to maintain the mindset that you're basically still keto, but you're simply adding healthy carbs.

It's crucial to focus on nurturing your body with *nutrition,* not getting into a good-bad relationship with carbs. Remember that healthy carbohydrates

- Fuel exercise performance
- Make muscle-building easier
- Help your body produce serotonin for overall happiness and sleep quality
- Increase thyroid hormone production (which means a faster metabolism)
- Provide a mountain of vitamins, minerals, and phytonutrients

Think about welcoming healthy carbs into your life in the same way you welcomed healthy fats during your keto phase. Optimizing your health is about gifting your body with the best possible nutrition. Remember that as you nurture your body with nutrient-dense carbohydrates during the reintroduction period.

It's ideal to ramp up your exercise intensity as you increase carbs so that you put those carbs to work and don't overfill your glycogen stores to the point of them spilling over into fat storage. I have provided a Four-Week Bring-Back-the-Carbs Training Plan with the Four-Week Bring-Back-the-Carbs Meal Plan to show you exactly how to do it. You don't have to work out to bring carbs back in, but it will enhance your results and get you feeling really good.

The training plan is geared toward intermediate to advanced gym-goers with five training days per week. If you are newer to training, I still want you to get the workouts in so that your body requires the increase in carbohydrates. That being said, please feel free to take it easy on the intensity. I want you to ease into things; I don't want you killing yourself in the gym until you're so sore that you can't perform well the next day.

To enhance your recovery, take 1 to 2 grams of vitamin C in the evening before bed. If you are experiencing muscle cramps, you might consider adding 2 grams a day of taurine as well. If you have injuries that limit you from doing the workouts, try to get in 10,000 steps a day or do another form of daily cardio that you enjoy.

Here's an overview of how your gradual reintroduction of carbohydrates and corresponding training plan will look:

Your Four-Week Bring-Back-the-Carbs Meal Plan Guidelines

First, note the following:

- You may add unlimited nonstarchy vegetables each week without tracking them if they do not cause bloating and gas. Depending on your gut microbial diversity, you may do extremely well with this approach, or you may get really bloated and experience digestive issues from adding in too much fiber at once. If it's the latter, cut back.

- You should prioritize starchy vegetables, fruit, and whole grains. You will not get the same beneficial effects if you choose processed carbs. You are human, and it might happen sometimes, but just know that your results won't be as positive if you choose those foods.

- Ideally, you should add the largest portion of carbs post-workout and combine it with protein.

How to configure your calories:

- For fat loss: Multiply your body weight in pounds by 10 to 12.
- For weight maintenance: Multiply your body weight in pounds by 13 to 15.
- For mass gain: Multiply your body weight in pounds by 16 to 18.

If you have a slower metabolism, have hypothyroidism, are perimenopausal, or are over age sixty, you'll likely need fewer calories, so play with your intake until you find a spot where you experience hunger at some point during the day, but it's tolerable, and you are slowly losing body fat.

How to set your macros:

WEEK 1:

- Protein: 40%
- Fat: 40%
- Carbs: 20%

WEEK 2:

- Protein: 40%
- Fat: 35%
- Carbs: 25%

WEEK 3:

- Protein: 40%
- Fat: 30%
- Carbs: 30%

WEEK 4:

- Protein: 40%
- Fat: 25%
- Carbs: 35%

A note on carbs: If you are not very active and don't have much muscle mass, you may not need as many carbs. So try this entire month as prescribed and take note of which amount of carbs feels optimal for you for your goals.

How to track your calories and macros:

I recommend downloading an app, such as MyFitnessPal. In MyFitnessPal, go to "More" in the bottom-right corner, choose "Goals," then choose "Calorie, Carbs, Protein & Fat Goals." Then set your calories and macros on the app according to the guidelines I have given here.

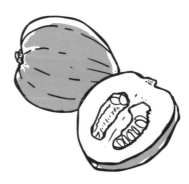

Here's an easy reference chart using 1,500 calories and 2,000 calories as examples:

		1,500-CALORIE PLAN			2,000-CALORIE PLAN		
		Protein	Fat	Carbs	Protein	Fat	Carbs
WEEK 1	Percentage of calories	40%	40%	20%	40%	40%	20%
	Grams	150g	67g	75g	200g	89g	100g
WEEK 2	Percentage of calories	40%	35%	25%	40%	35%	25%
	Grams	150g	58g	94g	200g	78g	125g
WEEK 3	Percentage of calories	40%	30%	30%	40%	30%	30%
	Grams	150g	50g	113g	200g	67g	150g
WEEK 4	Percentage of calories	40%	25%	35%	40%	25%	35%
	Grams	150g	42g	131g	200g	56g	175g

Your Four-Week Bring-Back-the-Carbs Training Plan Guidelines

- Monday: Lower Body + Cardio
- Tuesday: Chest, Back & Core + Cardio
- Wednesday: Lower Body + HIIT Circuit
- Thursday: Shoulders, Biceps & Triceps + Cardio
- Friday: Lower Body + Cardio
- Saturday: Upper/Lower Split + HIIT Cardio
- Sunday: Rest

For a metabolically flexible lifestyle, you can switch between keto and higher-carb days as often as you feel is necessary after you're fully keto-adapted and you've successfully reintroduced carbohydrates. For example, during the summer months, you may want to up your carb intake to match your higher activity levels; during the winter, you may want to do keto to accommodate lower activity levels. This approach enables you to fully enter into one mode or the other and complete a four-week training cycle to match your nutrition.

You can also experiment with the other metabolic flexibility approaches discussed in this chapter until you find the one that suits you best. Self-experimentation is a vital part of any health and fitness journey. Even if keto isn't a good fit for you long term, the metabolic flexibility that you create by training your body how to efficiently run on fat for fuel will do you huge favors in the long run. When your body can run equally efficiently on fat or carbs, weight maintenance is so much easier, which is the main reason I recommend keto.

Please remember throughout your journey that everyone is different. Some people absolutely thrive on keto, and others don't. Some feel way better when they eat carbs, and others do not. Some need to do keto for a year or more (especially in cases of diabetes, obesity, and therapeutic applications of the ketogenic diet), while others need to do it for only a month or two. It's important that you listen to your body and what feels most optimal for you while getting the results you want.

Please use the Four-Week Bring-Back-the-Carbs Meal Plan and Training Plan in Appendix C to experience what it's like to gradually reintroduce the right kinds of carbs after keto. You may swap out any carbohydrate source for another whole-food carbohydrate source from nature.

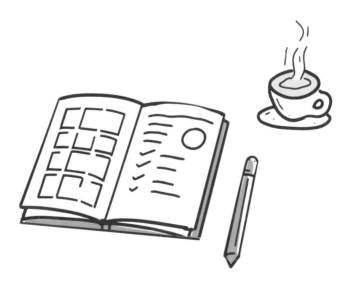

To sum it all up, my purpose in writing this book is to emphasize that while there is no one "right" nutritional approach for everyone, metabolic flexibility is a gift that all of us can create for our bodies! When we can eat according to actual hunger and match our nutrition to our exercise approach in an optimal way *for us,* everything gets easier.

I also wanted to get the point across that even as a ketogenic diet specialist, I do not feel keto is an optimal long-term nutritional approach for most people. Keto serves a purpose. It can be a powerful enhancer of the metabolism for people who are headed toward or have prediabetes, type 2 diabetes, obesity, or metabolic syndrome. It is also an incredible therapeutic intervention for many disease states. My hope is that we can all heal or optimize our bodies to the point that we can eat anything from nature and thrive!

I hope the research and strategies I have shared here will be valuable to you in your health journey. My goal is never to dogmatically prescribe anything to anyone, but rather to provide food for thought and strategies that you can try in an effort to find your sweet spot. And remember, as your body changes, your nutrition approach may need to change as well! Don't forget the story of my client Despina who lost nearly 100 pounds on keto. At the end of that weight loss, she was no longer in the same body. Her metabolism and exercise routine had completely changed! So be willing to make adjustments and try new approaches. As woo-woo as it may sound, I strongly encourage you to listen to your intuition. Ask your body what it needs and try doing what it asks you to do.

Lastly, be willing to change your approach when it no longer serves you. Just because something was the best solution at one point in your life doesn't mean it has to be that way forever. Diet variation is a natural part of the human experience. Once you are metabolically flexible, you should be able to thrive on a variety of nutritional approaches. Keep on experimenting and stay in each sweet spot for as long as you feel amazing, and then be willing to try something new.

Thank you so much for reading this book. I hope it has been helpful in your journey toward optimal health—there is nothing I wish more for you. Please come find me on Instagram (@coachtaragarrison) and let me know how your journey is going as you apply these methods!

Much love and health to you,

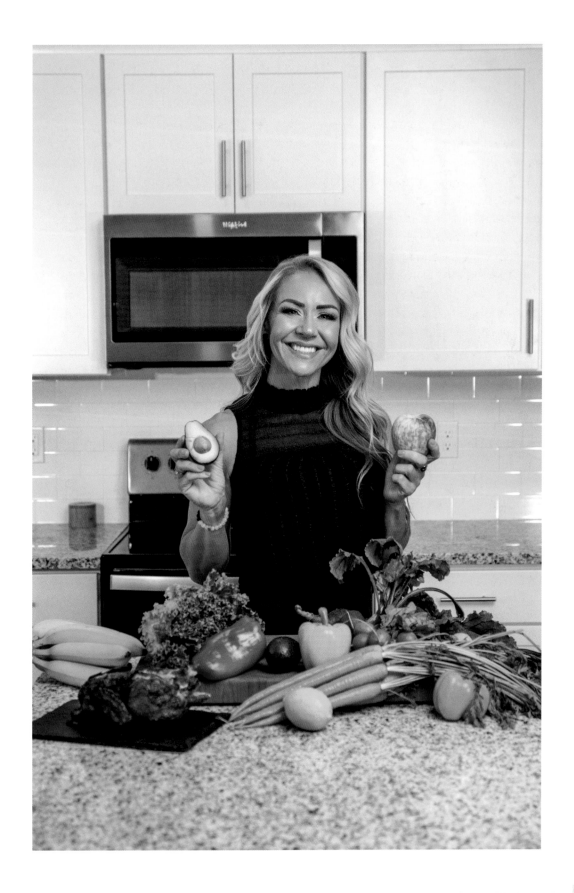

REFERENCES

1. Dylan A. Lowe et al., "Effects of Time-Restricted Eating on Weight Loss and Other Metabolic Parameters in Women and Men with Overweight and Obesity: The TREAT Randomized Clinical Trial," *JAMA Internal Medicine* 180, no. 1 (2020): 1491–9, https://doi.org/10.1001/jamainternmed.2020.4153.

2. Tatiana Moro et al., "Time-Restricted Eating Effects on Performance, Immune Function, and Body Composition in Elite Cyclists: A Randomized Controlled Trial," *Journal of the International Society of Sports Nutrition* 17, no. 1 (2020), accessed June 27, 2021, https://doi.org/10.1186/s12970-020-00396-z; Tatiana Moro et al., "Effects of Eight Weeks of Time-Restricted Feeding (16/8) on Basal Metabolism, Maximal Strength, Body Composition, Inflammation, and Cardiovascular Risk Factors in Resistance-Trained Males," *Journal of Translational Medicine* 14, no. 1 (2016): 290, https://doi.org/10.1186/s12967-016-1044-0.

3. Adrienne R. Barnosky et al., "Intermittent Fasting Vs. Daily Calorie Restriction for Type 2 Diabetes Prevention: A Review of Human Findings," *Translational Research* 164, no. 4 (2014): 302–11, https://doi.org/10.1016/j.trsl.2014.05.013.

4. Ruth E. Patterson and Dorothy D. Sears, "Metabolic Effects of Intermittent Fasting," *Annual Review of Nutrition* 37 (2017): 371–93, https://doi.org/10.1146/annurev-nutr-071816-064634.

5. Kulbhushan Tikoo et al., "Intermittent Fasting Prevents the Progression of Type 1 Diabetic Nephropathy in Rats and Changes the Expression of Sir2 and P53," *FEBS Letters* 581, no. 5 (2007): 1071–8, https://doi.org/10.1016/j.febslet.2007.02.006.

6. Mark P. Mattson and Ruiqian Wan, "Beneficial Effects of Intermittent Fasting and Caloric Restriction on the Cardiovascular and Cerebrovascular Systems," *Journal of Nutritional Biochemistry* 16, no. 3 (2005): 129–37, https://doi.org/10.1016/j.jnutbio.2004.12.007; James B. Johnson et al., "Alternate Day Calorie Restriction Improves Clinical Findings and Reduces Markers of Oxidative Stress and Inflammation in Overweight Adults with Moderate Asthma," *Free Radical Biology & Medicine* 42, no. 5 (2007): 665–74, https://doi.org/10.1016/j.freeradbiomed.2006.12.005; Fehime B. Aksungar, Aynur E. Topkaya, and Mahmut Akyildiz, "Interleukin-6, C-Reactive Protein and Biochemical Parameters During Prolonged Intermittent Fasting," *Annals of Nutrition & Metabolism* 51, no. 1 (2007): 88–95, https://doi.org/10.1159/000100954.

7. Fernanda R. de Azevedo, Dimas Ikeoka, and Bruno Caramelli, "Effects of Intermittent Fasting on Metabolism in Men," *Revista da Associacao Medica Brasileira* (1992) 59, no. 2 (2013): 167–73, https://doi.org/10.1016/j.ramb.2012.09.003; Rona Antoni et al., "The Effects of Intermittent Energy Restriction on Indices of Cardiometabolic Health," *Research in Endocrinology*, 2014 (2014): 1–24, https://doi.org/10.5171/2014.459119; Jaewon Lee et al., "Dietary Restriction Increases the Number of Newly Generated Neural Cells, and Induces BDNF Expression, in the Dentate Gyrus of Rats," *Journal of Molecular Neuroscience* 15, no. 2 (2000): 99–108, https://doi.org/10.1385/JMN:15:2:99.

8. Jaewon Lee, Kim B. Seroogy, and Mark P. Mattson, "Dietary Restriction Enhances Neurotrophin Expression and Neurogenesis in the Hippocampus of Adult Mice," *Journal of Neurochemistry* 80, no. 3 (2002), accessed June 27, 2021, https://doi.org/10.1046/j.0022-3042.2001.00747.x; C. L. Goodrick et al., "Differential Effects of Intermittent Feeding and Voluntary Exercise on Body Weight and Lifespan in Adult Rats," *Journal of Gerontology* 38, no. 1 (1983): 36–45, https://doi.org/10.1093/geronj/38.1.36.

9. Hiroshi Sogawa and Chiharu Kubo, "Influence of Short-Term Repeated Fasting on the Longevity of Female (NZB×NZW)F1 Mice," *Mechanisms of Ageing and Development* 115, 1–2 (2000): 61–71, https://doi.org/10.1016/S0047-6374(00)00109-3.

10. Rafael de Cabo and Mark P. Mattson, "Effects of Intermittent Fasting on Health, Aging, and Disease," *New England Journal of Medicine* 381, no. 26 (2019): 2541–51, https://doi.org/10.1056/NEJMra1905136.

11. Kim S. Stote et al., "A Controlled Trial of Reduced Meal Frequency Without Caloric Restriction in Healthy, Normal-Weight, Middle-Aged Adults," *American Journal of Clinical Nutrition* 85, no. 4 (2007): 981–8, https://doi.org/10.1093/ajcn/85.4.981.

12. Antonio Paoli et al., "The Influence of Meal Frequency and Timing on Health in Humans: The Role of Fasting," *Nutrients* 11, no. 4 (2019): 719, https://doi.org/10.3390/nu11040719.

13. Michael J. Ormsbee, Christopher W. Bach, and Daniel A. Baur, "Pre-Exercise Nutrition: The Role of Macronutrients, Modified Starches and Supplements on Metabolism and Endurance Performance," *Nutrients* 6, no. 5 (2014): 1782–808, https://doi.org/10.3390/nu6051782.

14. Adam Zajac et al., "The Effects of a Ketogenic Diet on Exercise Metabolism and Physical Performance in Off-Road Cyclists," *Nutrients* 6, no. 7 (2014): 2493–508, https://doi.org/10.3390/nu6072493.

15. Jichun Yang et al., "Leucine Metabolism in Regulation of Insulin Secretion from Pancreatic Beta Cells," *Nutrition Reviews* 68, no. 5 (2010): 270–9, https://doi.org/10.1111/j.1753-4887.2010.00282.x.

16. J. Langfort et al., "Effect of Low-Carbohydrate-Ketogenic Diet on Metabolic and Hormonal Responses to Graded Exercise in Men," *Journal of Physiology and Pharmacology* 47, no. 2 (1996): 361–71.

17. Jacob M. Wilson et al., "Effects of Ketogenic Dieting on Body Composition, Strength, Power, and Hormonal Profiles in Resistance Training Men," *Journal of Strength and Conditioning Research* 34, no. 12 (2020): 3463–74, doi: 10.1519/JSC.0000000000001935.

18. Lyle McDonald, "Carbing up on the Cyclical Ketogenic Diet," *Think Muscle,* accessed July 1, 2021, https://www.thinkmuscle.com/articles/mcdonald/carb-up-and-ketogenic-diet.htm.

19. J. L. Ivy et al., "Muscle Glycogen Synthesis After Exercise: Effect of Time of Carbohydrate Ingestion," *Journal of Applied Physiology* 64, no. 4 (1988): 1480–5, https://doi.org/10.1152/jappl.1988.64.4.1480.

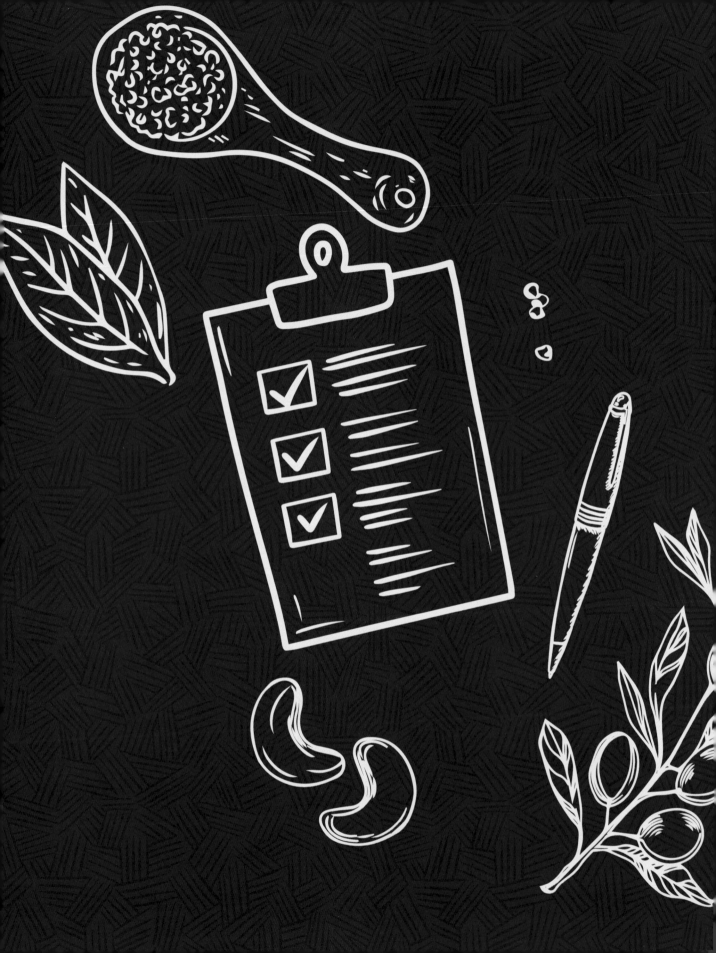

ONE-WEEK TARGETED KETOGENIC DIET PLAN

For more about targeted keto, please see pages 116 to 121.

ONE-WEEK TARGETED
KETOGENIC DIET
MEAL PLAN

For this plan, you will eat the same meals Monday through Wednesday and Thursday through Saturday to simplify meal prep and to avoid buying a ton of ingredients you won't use. Sunday has new recipes that are a little more fun for the weekend.

HOW TO CONFIGURE YOUR CALORIES:

- **For fat loss:** Multiply your body weight in pounds by 10. If you are not losing fat on this number of calories, or if the restriction is way too intense and you're absolutely starving, play with your calorie intake a little, moving it up or down until you find your sweet spot.

- **For maintenance:** Multiply your body weight in pounds by 13 or 14. You may have to play with your calorie intake a little, moving it up or down until you find your sweet spot.

- **For mass gain:** Multiply your body weight in pounds by 15 or 16. You may have to play with your calorie intake a little, moving it up or down until you find your sweet spot.

HOW TO SET YOUR MACROS:

On the days you work out:

- 55% fat

- 30% protein

- 15% carbs (mostly in the post-workout window)

Example menus are set at 1,500 and 2,000 calories per day. Use the formulas above to calculate your own calories and macros.

		1,500-CALORIE PLAN		2,000-CALORIE PLAN	
MONDAY to WEDNESDAY	**Breakfast:** Carrot Cake Protein Smoothie *(page 139)* **Lunch:** Pan-Seared Salmon with Tomato Salad* *(page 140)* **Dinner:** Garlic Zucchini Frittata *(page 142)*	Calories:	**1,508**	Calories:	**2,024**
		Protein:	**120g**	Protein:	**171g**
		Carbs:	**59g**	Carbs:	**74g**
		Fat:	**88g**	Fat:	**116g**
THURSDAY to SATURDAY	**Breakfast:** Raspberry Protein Smoothie *(page 143)* **Lunch:** Smoky Chicken Thighs & Creamed Spinach* *(page 144)* **Dinner:** Broccoli & Feta Frittata *(page 146)*	Calories:	**1,534**	Calories:	**2,040**
		Protein:	**112g**	Protein:	**155g**
		Carbs:	**51g**	Carbs:	**58g**
		Fat:	**98g**	Fat:	**132g**
SUNDAY	**Breakfast:** Matcha Protein Smoothie* *(page 147)* **Lunch:** Zesty Chicken & Grapefruit Salad *(page 148)* **Dinner:** Cheese Crackers & Guacamole *(page 150)*	Calories:	**1,533**	Calories:	**1,973**
		Protein:	**111g**	Protein:	**154g**
		Carbs:	**54g**	Carbs:	**76g**
		Fat:	**97g**	Fat:	**117g**

If you are following the 2,000-Calorie Plan, you will eat a double portion of this meal.

Please note that calories and macro grams can vary depending on the app you are using to track, so if you are logging your meals in an app and the numbers don't match up perfectly with the numbers shown in this book, don't worry. This is normal. It will be close enough to get you the results you need.

TARGETED KETO
SHOPPING LIST

*Additional quantities for the 2,000-Calorie Plan are marked with an asterisk.

MEAT, EGGS & DAIRY:

Boneless, skinless chicken breast, 4½ ounces (about 1 small breast)

Boneless, skinless chicken thighs, 15 ounces (*add 15 ounces)

Eggs, 21 large

Feta cheese, 6 ounces

Greek yogurt, plain nonfat, 43 ounces

Heavy cream, 4½ tablespoons (3 ounces) (*add 4½ tablespoons [3 ounces])

Salmon fillets, 1½ pounds (*add 1½ pounds)

White cheddar cheese, 3 ounces

FRESH PRODUCE:

Arugula, 3 cups (2.1 ounces)

Avocado, 1 medium (*add 1)

Bananas, 2 medium

Basil, 1 bunch

Broccoli, 9 ounces (1 head)

Carrots, 5 medium

Cherry tomatoes, 6 cups (about 2⅔ pounds) (*add 6 cups)

Cilantro, 1 bunch

Garlic, 1 head

Ginger root, 1

Grapefruit, 1

Lemons, 2

Lime, 1

Parsley, 1 bunch

Raspberries, 3 cups

Spinach, 18 ounces (*add 18 ounces)

Zucchini, 4 medium

PANTRY ITEMS:

Almond butter, 6 tablespoons (3 ounces)

Almond milk, unsweetened, 10 ounces (*add 10 ounces)

Balsamic vinegar, 3 tablespoons (*add 3 tablespoons)

Extra-virgin olive oil, 10 ounces (*add 3 ounces)

Matcha powder, 1 teaspoon

Nutritional yeast, 2 tablespoons

Powdered stevia, 4½ teaspoons (*add ½ teaspoon)

Whey protein powder, 10½ ounces (*add 1½ ounces)

SPICES & SEEDS:

Black peppercorns

Chia seeds, ½ cup (4 ounces)

Salt

Smoked paprika

CARROT CAKE
PROTEIN SMOOTHIE

½ cup plain nonfat Greek yogurt

2 ounces whey protein powder

1½ tablespoons chia seeds

1½ medium carrots, roughly chopped

½ medium banana

1 teaspoon grated ginger

¼ teaspoon powdered stevia

Whiz all the ingredients in a blender. Add water as needed to achieve the desired consistency. Pour into a tall glass and serve immediately.

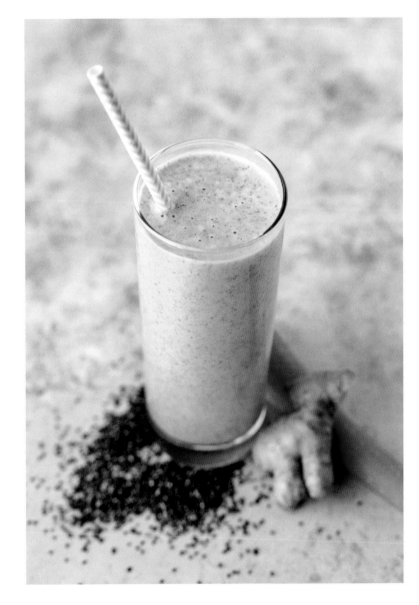

CALORIES:	PROTEIN:	CARBS:	FAT:
486	53g	37g	14g

PAN-SEARED SALMON
WITH TOMATO SALAD

MON
TO
WED

FOR 1,500-CALORIE PLAN:

1 tablespoon extra-virgin olive oil, divided

2 (4-ounce) salmon fillets

½ teaspoon salt

½ teaspoon ground black pepper

2 cups cherry tomatoes, halved

1 clove garlic, minced

1 tablespoon balsamic vinegar

4 sprigs fresh basil, for garnish

FOR 2,000-CALORIE PLAN:

2 tablespoons extra-virgin olive oil, divided

4 (4-ounce) salmon fillets

1 teaspoon salt

1 teaspoon ground black pepper

4 cups cherry tomatoes, halved

2 cloves garlic, minced

2 tablespoons balsamic vinegar

8 sprigs fresh basil, for garnish

1. Heat half of the oil in a skillet over medium heat, rotating the skillet to coat the bottom with the oil. Season the salmon fillets on both sides with the salt and pepper. When the oil is hot, carefully place the salmon skin side down in the pan and cook until crispy, 5 to 7 minutes. Carefully turn the fillets over, cover the skillet with a lid, reduce the heat to medium-low, and cook until the fish is opaque and flakes easily, about 10 more minutes. Transfer to a serving plate.

2. Meanwhile, in a medium bowl, toss together the tomatoes, garlic, vinegar, and remaining oil. Season with salt and pepper to taste. Spoon the tomato salad over the salmon and garnish with the basil.

1,500-CALORIE PLAN:

CALORIES:	PROTEIN:	CARBS:	FAT:
516	51g	15g	28g

2,000-CALORIE PLAN:

CALORIES:	PROTEIN:	CARBS:	FAT:
1,032	102g	30g	56g

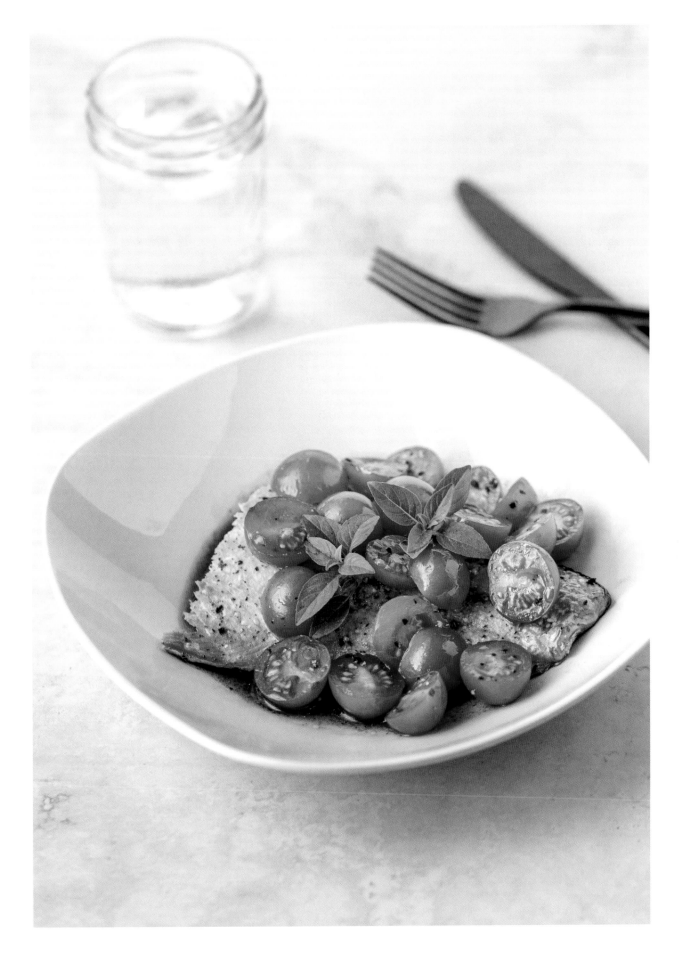

MON
TO
WED

GARLIC ZUCCHINI
FRITTATA

2 tablespoons extra-virgin olive oil

1 clove garlic, minced

1 cup thin quarter slices zucchini

1 large egg

3 large egg yolks

½ teaspoon salt

½ teaspoon ground black pepper

Finely chopped fresh parsley, for garnish

1. Heat the oil in a small skillet over medium heat. Add the garlic and cook, stirring constantly, until lightly browned, about 30 seconds. Add the zucchini and cook, stirring often, until soft, 5 to 7 minutes.

2. In a small bowl, beat the egg and egg yolks with a fork just until well blended. Stir in the salt and pepper and pour into the skillet. Cover with a lid, reduce the heat to low, and cook until the eggs are set in the center, about 5 minutes. Serve garnished with parsley.

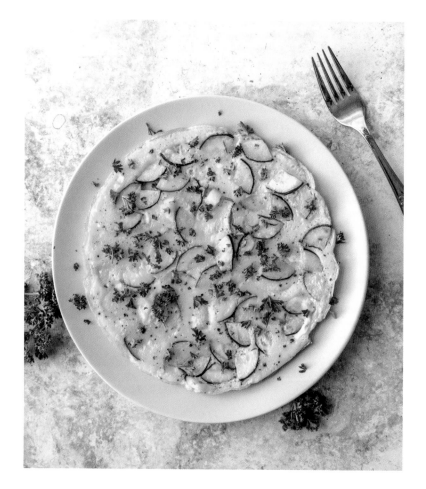

CALORIES:	PROTEIN:	CARBS:	FAT:
506	16g	7g	46g

RASPBERRY
PROTEIN SMOOTHIE

1 cup plain nonfat Greek
yogurt

1 cup raspberries

2 tablespoons almond butter

1 tablespoon chia seeds

1 ounce whey protein powder

1 teaspoon powdered stevia

Whiz all the ingredients in a blender. Add water as needed to achieve the desired consistency. Pour into a tall glass and serve immediately.

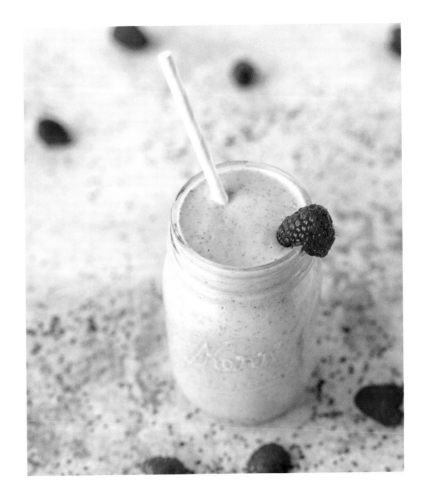

CALORIES:	PROTEIN:	CARBS:	FAT:
516	41g	34g	24g

SMOKY CHICKEN THIGHS & CREAMED SPINACH

THU TO SAT

FOR 1,500-CALORIE PLAN:

1½ tablespoons extra-virgin olive oil, divided

1 teaspoon smoked paprika

½ teaspoon salt

½ teaspoon ground black pepper

5 ounces boneless, skinless chicken thighs

5 ounces fresh spinach

1½ tablespoons heavy cream

Finely chopped fresh parsley, for garnish

FOR 2,000-CALORIE PLAN:

3 tablespoons extra-virgin olive oil, divided

2 teaspoons smoked paprika

1 teaspoon salt

1 teaspoon ground black pepper

10 ounces boneless, skinless chicken thighs

10 ounces fresh spinach

3 tablespoons heavy cream

Finely chopped fresh parsley, for garnish

1. Heat half of the oil in a medium skillet over medium-high heat. Sprinkle the paprika, salt, and pepper on the chicken thighs and massage well to distribute the seasonings evenly. Brown the chicken lightly on both sides. Cover with a lid, reduce the heat to medium-low, and cook until the chicken is cooked through in the center (use two forks to separate the meat), about 15 minutes.

2. Heat the rest of the oil in a small skillet over medium heat. Add the spinach and cook until wilted, about 1 minute. Pour in the cream, season with salt and pepper to taste, and mix well.

3. Serve the chicken on the creamed spinach and garnish with parsley.

1,500-CALORIE PLAN:

CALORIES:	PROTEIN:	CARBS:	FAT:
506	43g	7g	34g

2,000-CALORIE PLAN:

CALORIES:	PROTEIN:	CARBS:	FAT:
1,012	86g	14g	68g

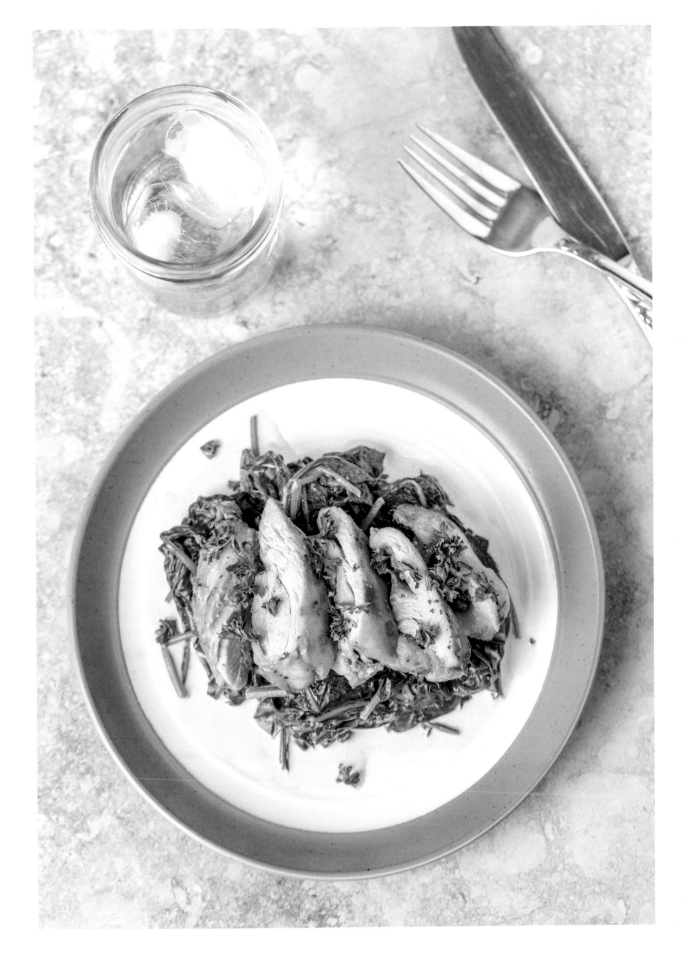

BROCCOLI &
FETA FRITTATA

1 tablespoon extra-virgin olive oil

3 ounces broccoli, finely chopped

3 large eggs

¼ teaspoon salt

¼ teaspoon ground black pepper

2 ounces feta cheese, drained

1. Heat the oil in a medium skillet over medium heat. Add the broccoli and cook until slightly softened, about 2 minutes.

2. In a small bowl, beat the eggs with a fork just until well blended, then season with the salt and pepper.

3. Stir the feta into the broccoli, then pour the egg mixture into the skillet. Cover with a lid, reduce the heat to low, and cook until the eggs are firm, about 10 minutes.

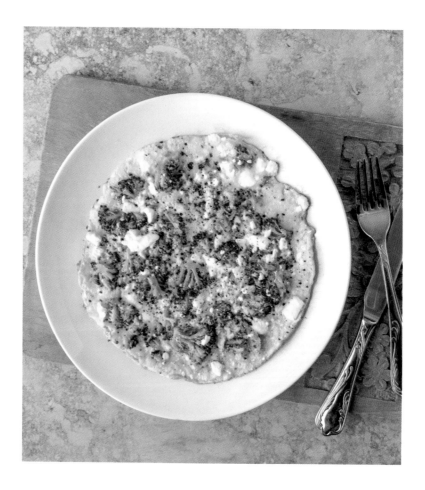

CALORIES:	PROTEIN:	CARBS:	FAT:
512	28g	10g	40g

MATCHA
PROTEIN SMOOTHIE

FOR 1,500-CALORIE PLAN:

3 ounces fresh spinach

½ medium avocado, peeled and pitted

1½ ounces whey protein powder

1 teaspoon matcha powder

1¼ cups unsweetened almond milk

½ teaspoon liquid or powdered stevia

FOR 2,000-CALORIE PLAN:

6 ounces fresh spinach

1 medium avocado, halved, peeled, and pitted

3 ounces whey protein powder

2 teaspoons matcha powder

2½ cups unsweetened almond milk

1 teaspoon liquid or powdered stevia

Whiz all the ingredients in a blender. Pour into a tall glass and serve immediately.

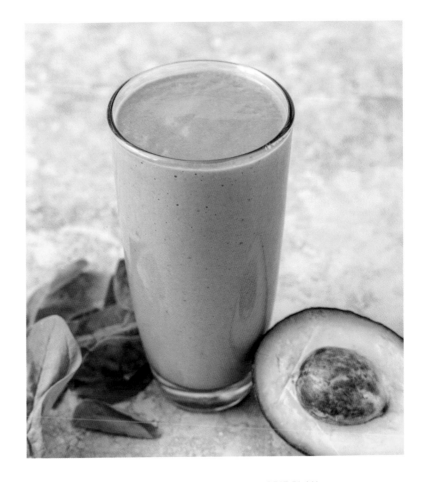

1,500-CALORIE PLAN:			
CALORIES:	PROTEIN:	CARBS:	FAT:
440	43g	22g	20g

2,000-CALORIE PLAN:			
CALORIES:	PROTEIN:	CARBS:	FAT:
880	86g	44g	40g

SHORT-TERM KETO

SUN

ZESTY CHICKEN & GRAPEFRUIT SALAD

4½ ounces boneless, skinless chicken breast (about 1 small breast)

½ teaspoon salt, divided

½ teaspoon ground black pepper, divided

2 tablespoons extra-virgin olive oil, divided

3 cups arugula

2 tablespoons nutritional yeast, plus more for garnish

¼ cup lemon juice

1 tablespoon plain nonfat Greek yogurt

1½ ounces grapefruit sections, cut into chunks, for garnish

Finely chopped fresh herbs of choice, for garnish

1. Preheat a large skillet over medium-high heat. Rub the chicken with ¼ teaspoon of the salt and ¼ teaspoon of the pepper. Coat the bottom of the skillet with 1 tablespoon of the oil, add the seasoned chicken, and cook for 2 to 3 minutes on each side, until cooked through. Remove the pan from the heat and allow the chicken to cool slightly.

2. Arrange the arugula in a serving bowl. When the chicken is cool enough to handle, cut it against the grain into ½-inch slices.

3. Make the dressing: In a small bowl, stir together the remaining tablespoon of oil, the nutritional yeast, lemon juice, yogurt, remaining ¼ teaspoon of salt, and remaining ¼ teaspoon of pepper.

4. Drizzle the dressing over the arugula and top with the chicken, grapefruit chunks, herbs, and a sprinkling of nutritional yeast.

CALORIES:	PROTEIN:	CARBS:	FAT:
520	52g	15g	28g

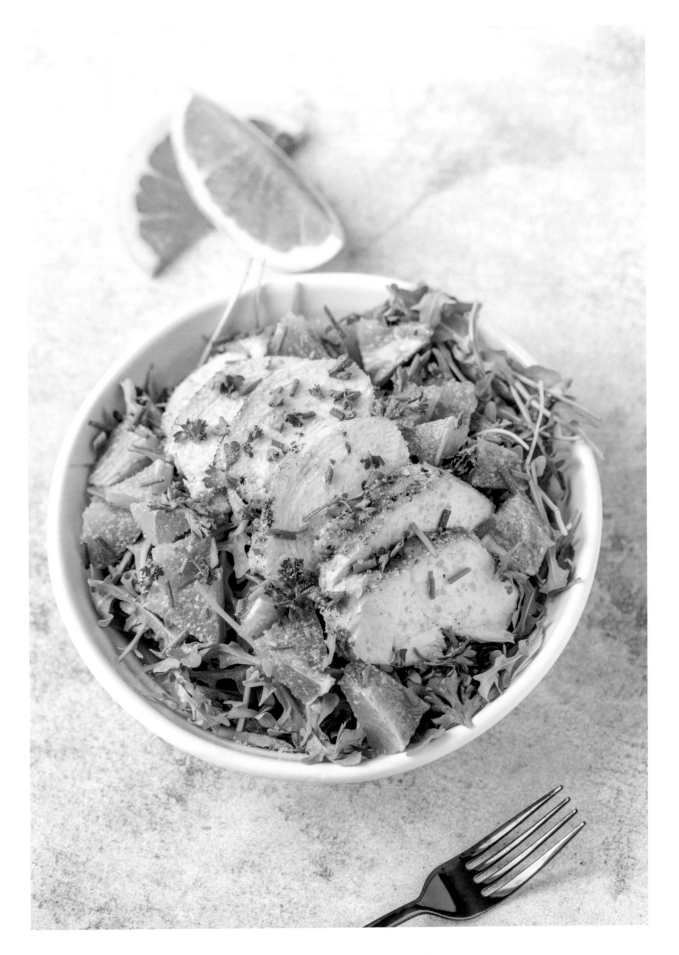

SUN

GUACAMOLE &
CHEESE CRACKERS

3 ounces white cheddar cheese, shredded

½ medium avocado, peeled and pitted

2 tablespoons finely chopped fresh cilantro, plus extra leaves for garnish

1 tablespoon lime juice

1 tablespoon extra-virgin olive oil

¼ teaspoon salt

¼ teaspoon ground black pepper

1. Preheat the oven to 350°F. Line a baking sheet with parchment paper.

2. Divide the cheese into three equal portions and carefully spoon each portion into a pile on the prepared baking sheet. Bake until golden brown, about 12 minutes. Remove the sheet from the oven and let the crackers cool completely before removing with a spatula to a serving plate.

3. Scoop the avocado flesh into a small bowl. Use a fork to break it up and stir in the cilantro, lime juice, and olive oil. Season with the salt and pepper.

4. Top the cheese crackers with the guacamole and garnish with cilantro.

CALORIES:	PROTEIN:	CARBS:	FAT:
573	16g	17g	49g

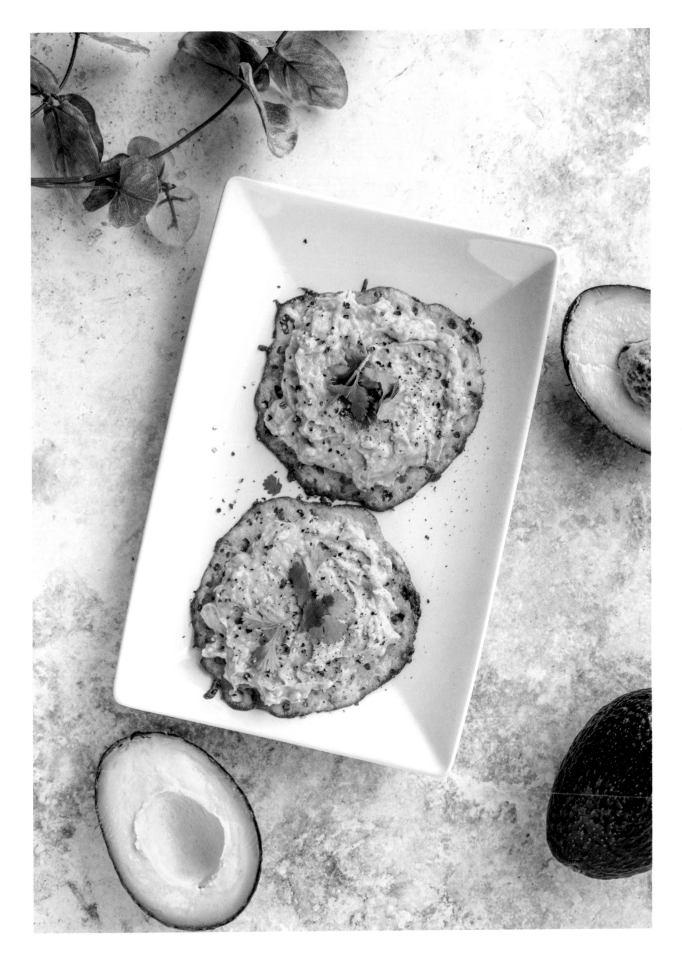

ONE-WEEK TARGETED
KETOGENIC DIET TRAINING PLAN

Monday	Lower Body Training
Tuesday	Back, Chest, and Core + Cardio
Wednesday	High-Intensity Interval Training: Functional Circuit
Thursday	Lower Body Training
Friday	Shoulders, Triceps, Biceps, and Core + Cardio
Saturday	High-Intensity Interval Training: Cardio
Sunday	Upper/Lower Body Training

Please visit my YouTube channel for exercise demo videos: YouTube.com/coachtaragarrison.

UNDERSTANDING YOUR TRAINING PLAN

In this plan, I give you a full week of workouts, so you have options. However, you do not need to train all seven days. On the days you take off from the gym or just walk, simply eat a standard ketogenic diet, with macros of approximately 65 to 70 percent fat, 25 to 30 percent protein, and 5 percent carbs, or carbs low enough that you stay in ketosis.

MONDAY: LOWER BODY TRAINING

Warm up on the cardio machine of your choice for 5 to 10 minutes, then complete the following sequence:

1. **Bodyweight Walking Lunges:** 1 set of 20 (10/leg). Focus on form. Your front heel must make contact with the floor with each lunge. Your back knee will hover just above the floor without actually touching it. Rest for 30 seconds after the set.

2. **Walking Lunges with dumbbells at sides:** 3 sets of 20 (10/leg). Increase the weight with each set. Rest for 45 to 60 seconds between sets.

3. **Step-Ups with dumbbells at sides:** 3 sets of 20 (10/leg). Complete 10 step-ups on one leg and then switch legs. Make sure your entire foot (including your heel) is making contact with the platform or box. The platform or box should be at a height that creates a 90-degree angle with your leg when you step onto it. Rest for 45 to 60 seconds between sets.

4. **Goblet Squats:** 3 sets of 15. Increase the weight with each set, and do not pause at the top or bottom. Keep your knees outside of your big toes. Rest for 45 to 60 seconds between sets.

5. **Dumbbell Romanian Deadlifts:** 3 sets of 12. Hold one dumbbell in each hand and keep them close to your legs during the movement. Increase the weight with each set. Rest for 45 to 60 seconds between sets.

6. **Barbell or Dumbbell Hip Thrusts:** 4 sets of 15. Do this exercise with a barbell (padded around the shaft to protect your hip bones) if you have access to one. Squeeze your glutes at the top of the thrust. Increase the weight with each set. Rest for 60 seconds between sets.

7. **Dumbbell Leg Curls:** 3 sets of 12. Increase the weight with each set. Rest for 45 to 60 seconds between sets.

8. **Seated or Standing Calf Raises:** 3 sets of 30 reps broken down as follows: 10 slow, 10 quick pulses at the top, 10 regular. On the first 10 reps, go slowly on the way down for a count of five and then explode into the peak contraction for a count of one. Hold at the top for a count of one before slowly lowering back down for a count of five. The set of 10 pulses will be as quick as possible, and the last 10 reps can be at any speed that feels natural to you. Using a machine is ideal for this exercise, but you can do bodyweight calf raises or hold dumbbells at your sides if that's what's available to you. Rest for 60 seconds between sets.

TUESDAY: BACK, CHEST, AND CORE + CARDIO

Warm up on the cardio machine of your choice for 5 to 10 minutes. Then complete the following sequence, increasing the weight with each set and resting for 45 to 60 seconds after each set.

1. Lat Pulldowns: 3 sets of 12

2. Cable Chest Flies: 3 sets of 12

3. Cable Chops for Abs: 3 sets of 24 (12/side)

4. Seated Cable Rows: 3 sets of 12

5. Barbell Bench Presses: 3 sets of 12

6. Cable Lifts for Abs: 3 sets of 24 (12/side)

Finish with 20 minutes of cardio intervals using the method of your choice. Warm up for 5 minutes, then alternate with this pattern: fast pace (doesn't need to be a sprint, just a push) for 1 minute followed by a comfortable pace for 2 minutes for the remaining 15 minutes.

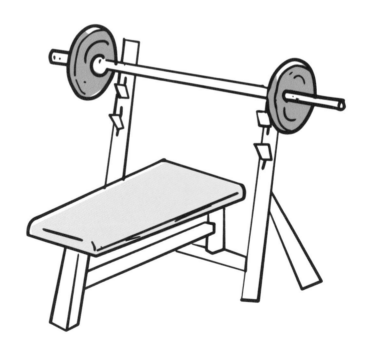

WEDNESDAY: HIGH-INTENSITY INTERVAL TRAINING: FUNCTIONAL CIRCUIT

Warm up on the cardio machine of your choice for 5 to 10 minutes.

Functional HIIT Circuit: You will perform each exercise for 30 seconds, rest for 30 seconds, and then move on to the next exercise. After you have completed all six exercises, rest for 2 minutes, and then repeat the entire circuit two more times. You will do a total of three rounds. Go hard or go home, baby! This entire workout is only 21 minutes long! When time goes down, intensity goes up. Get in, get it done, and get out.

1. Sled Pushes or "Deadmill" (run on a treadmill with it turned off while holding on to the handles)
2. Walking Push-Ups
3. Box Jumps (or jump rope if you can't box jump safely)
4. Battle Ropes or Medicine Ball Slams with a lot of power
5. Sprint (or Sled Pushes again if you can't sprint safely)
6. Wall Balls with medicine ball

THURSDAY: LOWER BODY TRAINING

Warm up on the cardio machine of your choice for 5 minutes. Then complete the following sequence, increasing the weight with each set and resting for 45 to 60 seconds after each set.

1. Lying Hamstring Curls: 3 sets of 12
2. Leg Extensions: 3 sets of 12
3. Standing Calf Raises: 3 sets of 12
4. 45-Degree Hip Extensions: 3 sets of 12
5. Dumbbell Split Squats or Rear Foot Elevated Dumbbell Split Squats (if you need it to be harder): 3 sets of 20 (10/leg)
6. Seated Calf Raises: 3 sets of 12

FRIDAY: SHOULDERS, TRICEPS, BICEPS, AND CORE + CARDIO

Warm up on the cardio machine of your choice for 5 to 10 minutes. Then complete the following sequence, resting for 45 to 60 seconds after each set.

1. Seated Overhead Dumbbell Presses: 3 sets of 12. Increase the weight with each set.

2. Dumbbell Lateral Raises: 3 sets of 12. On the way down, your movement should be slow and controlled. Don't rest at the bottom.

3. Triceps Kickbacks: 3 sets of 24 to 30 (12 to 15/arm). Make sure the weight is heavy enough to be challenging but not so heavy that you can't contract your triceps all the way. Increase the weight with each set.

4. Triceps Rope Extensions: 3 sets of 12. Increase the weight each set.

5. Biceps 21s: 3 sets of 7 lower half of a biceps curl, 7 upper half of a biceps curl, and 7 full-range biceps curls.

6. Biceps Kettlebell Triset of Terror: 3 total sets. While sitting on an incline bench, do 10 of each variation: 45-degree biceps curls with kettlebell held straight out, 10 hammer curls, and 10 underhand grip regular biceps curls.

Finish with 20 minutes of cardio intervals using the method of your choice. Warm up for 5 minutes, then alternate with this pattern: fast pace (doesn't need to be a sprint, just a push) for 1 minute followed by a comfortable pace for 2 minutes for the remaining 15 minutes.

SATURDAY: HIGH-INTENSITY INTERVAL TRAINING: CARDIO

Choose your preferred cardio method. I recommend the stair mill for many people. If you are an experienced runner, you may run, but I don't recommend it if running is not a normal exercise for you. I don't want you to get injured. A bike or rowing machine works as well. The elliptical is the option I recommend least often because I just don't see people getting good results from it. However, if that's all you have or you need to use one because of injuries, that's fine. Walking is not intense enough. This is a high-heart-rate training session on the high-intensity intervals.

Workout Duration: 30 minutes

Warm up for 5 minutes. Do 30 seconds of an all-out sprint followed by 2 minutes of work at a comfortable pace. Repeat this pattern of 30-second sprint and 2 minutes of comfortable pace for the remaining 25 minutes.

SUNDAY: UPPER/LOWER BODY TRAINING

Warm up on the cardio machine of your choice for 5 to 10 minutes, then complete the following sequence:

1. **Barbell or Dumbbell Push Presses:** 3 sets of 8. Increase the weight with each set. Rest for 45 to 60 seconds between sets.

2. **Double Kettlebell Front Squats:** 3 sets of 12. Increase the weight with each set. Rest for 60 seconds between sets.

3. **Dumbbell Upright Rows:** 3 sets of 12. Increase the weight with each set. Rest for 45 to 60 seconds between sets.

4. **Single-Leg Deadlifts:** 3 sets of 24 (12/leg). You can extend your opposite arm to support your balance. Keep the dumbbell close to your shin. Increase the weight with each set. Rest for 45 to 60 seconds between sets.

5. **Hammer Curls:** 3 sets of 12. Increase the weight with each set. Rest for 45 to 60 seconds between sets.

6. **45-Degree Hip Extensions:** 3 sets of 15. Use the back extension machine, but let your back round so you use your glutes. You can hold a plate to your chest if you need extra weight. If you don't have a back extension machine, do dumbbell or barbell hip thrusts instead. Rest for 60 seconds between sets.

7. **Triceps Rope Cable Extensions:** 3 sets of 15. If you don't have cables, do skull crushers. Increase the weight with each set. Rest for 45 to 60 seconds between sets.

8. **Seated or Standing Calf Raises:** 3 sets of 25. If you don't have a machine, do bodyweight calf raises or hold dumbbells at your sides. Rest for 45 to 60 seconds between sets.

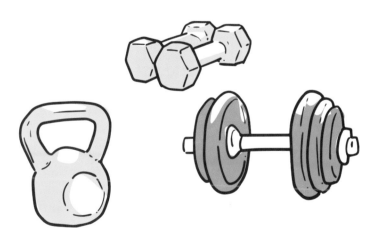

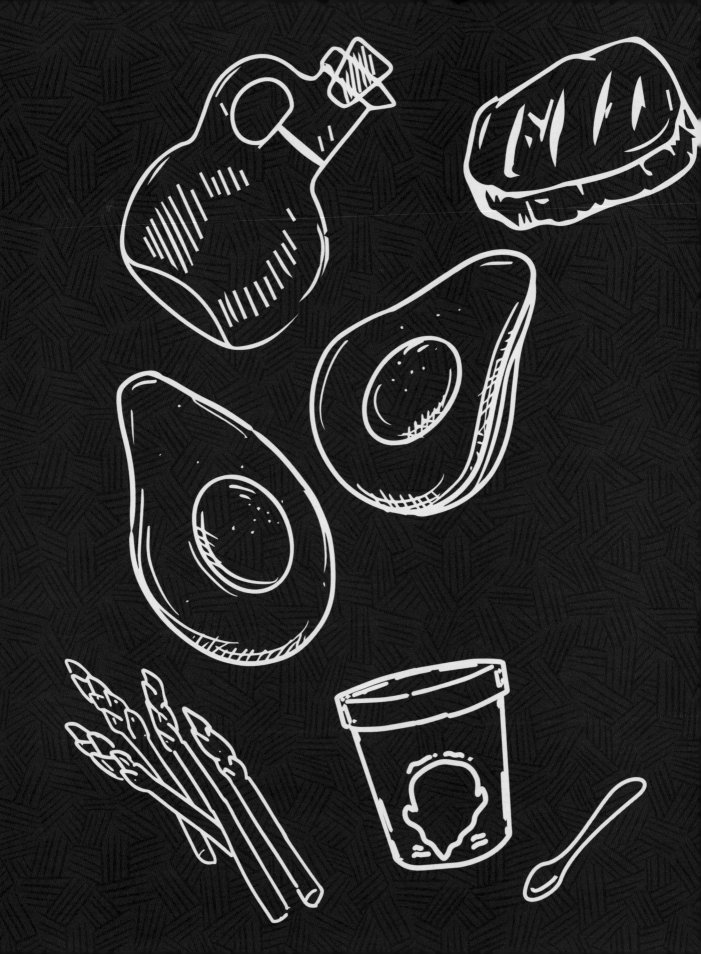

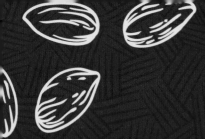

APPENDIX B

ONE-WEEK CYCLICAL KETOGENIC DIET PLAN

For more about cyclical keto, please see pages 122 to 124.

ONE-WEEK CYCLICAL
KETOGENIC DIET
MEAL PLAN

For this plan, you will eat the same meals Monday through Thursday. Then you will have different meals on Friday and Saturday, as your macro targets will be different on those days. On Sunday, you will fast to get back into ketosis quickly. You can fast the entire day or break your fast with the ketogenic dinner of your choice.

HOW TO CONFIGURE YOUR CALORIES:

- **For fat loss:** Multiply your body weight in pounds by 10. If you are not losing fat on this number of calories, or the restriction is way too intense and you're absolutely starving, move your calorie intake up or down a little until you find your sweet spot.

- **For maintenance:** Multiply your body weight in pounds by 13 or 14. You may have to play with your calorie intake a little, moving it up or down until you find your sweet spot.

- **For mass gain:** Multiply your body weight in pounds by 15 or 16. You may have to play with your calorie intake a little, moving it up or down until you find your sweet spot.

HOW TO SET YOUR MACROS:

- **Monday–Thursday (keto):** 65% fat, 30% protein, 5% carbs
- **Friday (high-carb):** 15% fat, 20% protein, 65% carbs
- **Saturday (high-carb):** 20% fat, 30% protein, 50% carbs
- **Sunday:** Fast to get back into ketosis. You can either fast the entire day or break your fast at dinner with a ketogenic meal.

Example menus are set at 1,500 and 2,000 calories per day. Use the formulas above to calculate your own calories and macros.

		1,500-CALORIE PLAN		2,000-CALORIE PLAN	
MONDAY to THURSDAY	**Breakfast:** Poached Eggs & Avocado *(page 164)* **Lunch:** Baked Lemon Salmon & Asparagus* *(page 166)* **Dinner:** Swedish Meatballs & Arugula *(page 168)*	Calories:	**1,470**	Calories:	**1,944**
		Protein:	**106g**	Protein:	**153g**
		Carbs:	**23g**	Carbs:	**27g**
		Fat:	**106g**	Fat:	**136g**
FRIDAY	**Breakfast:** Sweet Potato Egg White Scramble *(page 170)* **Lunch:** Baked Butternut Squash with Orange & Raisins *(page 171)* **Dinner:** Aromatic Rice & Chicken* *(page 172)*	Calories:	**1,511**	Calories:	**2,003**
		Protein:	**78g**	Protein:	**116g**
		Carbs:	**248g**	Carbs:	**324g**
		Fat:	**23g**	Fat:	**27g**
SATURDAY	**Breakfast:** Garlic Rice–Stuffed Portobello Mushrooms* *(page 174)* **Lunch:** Pulled Pork Tacos with Potatoes *(page 176)* **Dinner:** Baked Turkey & Apples *(page 177)*	Calories:	**1,482**	Calories:	**2,009**
		Protein:	**121g**	Protein:	**143g**
		Carbs:	**182g**	Carbs:	**276g**
		Fat:	**30g**	Fat:	**37g**
SUNDAY		**Fast**			

*If you are following the 2,000-Calorie Plan, you will eat a double portion of this meal.

Instructions for slow-cooking the pork for Saturday:

Rub 10 ounces boneless pork shoulder with salt and pepper, place in a slow cooker, and cook on low for 4 hours. Remove the pork from the pot and shred using two forks.

CYCLICAL KETO
SHOPPING LIST

*Additional quantities for the 2,000-Calorie Plan are marked with an asterisk.

MEAT, EGGS & DAIRY:

Boneless, skinless chicken breast, 8 ounces (*add 8 ounces)

Boneless, skinless turkey breast, 9 ounces

Eggs, 20 large

Egg whites, 7 large, or 14 tablespoons liquid egg whites

Ground beef, 12 ounces

Ground pork, 6 ounces

Heavy cream, 1 cup (8 ounces)

Low-fat yogurt, plain, 3½ ounces

Pork shoulder, lean, 7½ ounces

Salmon fillets, 2 pounds (*add 2 pounds)

Sour cream, 1 cup (8 ounces)

FRESH PRODUCE:

Arugula, 8½ cups (6 ounces)

Asparagus, 12 ounces (*add 12 ounces)

Avocados, 4 medium

Butternut squash, 5 cups cubed (about 3½ pounds)

Cilantro, 1 bunch

Fuji apple, 8 ounces (about 1 large)

Garlic, 1 head

Lemons, 2 (*add 2)

Lime, 1

Orange, 1 medium

Parsley, 1 bunch

Portobello mushrooms, 4 large (about 4 ounces each) (*add 4 large mushrooms)

Romaine lettuce, 3 large leaves

Sweet potatoes, 2 medium

Thyme, 1 bunch

Tomato, 1 medium

Waxy potatoes, 2 medium

Yellow or white onion, 1 medium

PANTRY ITEMS:

Basmati rice, 1 cup (*add 1 cup)

Beef stock, 2 cups

Blanched almond flour, ½ cup

Extra-virgin olive oil, ⅜ cup

Maple syrup, 1 tablespoon

Raisins, 3 ounces

Whey protein powder, 4 ounces

Worcestershire sauce, 4 teaspoons

SPICES & SEEDS:

Black peppercorns

Cardamom pods

Coarse salt

Fine salt

Ground allspice

Ground cinnamon

Ground nutmeg

Star anise pods

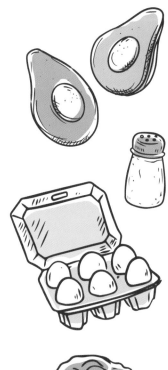

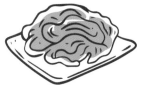

MON
TO
THU

POACHED EGGS &
AVOCADO

4 large eggs

1 medium avocado, halved

Salt and cracked black pepper

Fresh thyme leaves, for garnish (optional)

1. Poach the eggs: Bring at least 2 inches of water to a boil in a large saucepan over high heat, then reduce the heat to a simmer.

2. Crack an egg into a bowl or onto a saucer; this makes it easier to slide the egg into the pan. If there is any very runny white surrounding the thicker white, tip it away.

3. Stir the water in the saucepan to create a gentle whirlpool to help the egg white wrap around the yolk, then gently drop the egg into the center of the whirlpool. Make sure the heat is low enough not to throw the egg around; there should be only small bubbles rising. Cook the egg for 3 to 4 minutes, or until the white is set.

4. Lift the egg out of the water with a slotted spoon and lay it on a paper towel to drain. Repeat this process with the remaining eggs.

5. If desired, peel, pit, and slice the avocado. Serve the poached eggs with the avocado on the side. Season with a pinch each of salt and pepper and garnish with thyme, if desired.

CALORIES:	PROTEIN:	CARBS:	FAT:
524	28g	13g	40g

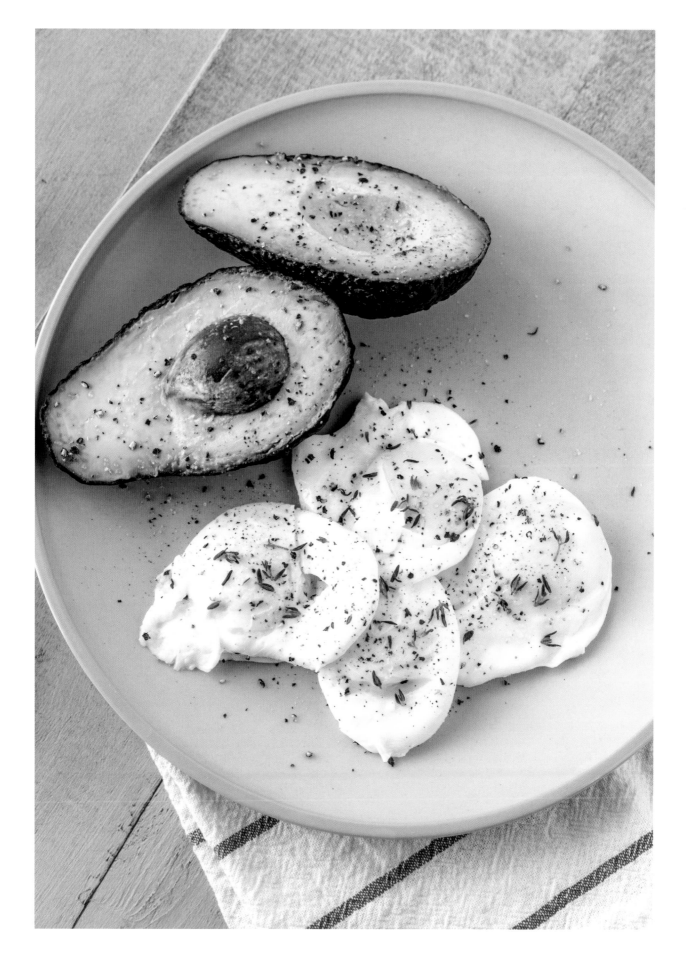

LUNCH

BAKED LEMON SALMON & ASPARAGUS

MON
TO
THU

FOR 1,500-CALORIE PLAN:

2 (4-ounce) salmon fillets

3 ounces trimmed asparagus

1 tablespoon lemon juice

1 clove garlic, minced

½ teaspoon salt

½ teaspoon ground black pepper

Lemon slices, for garnish

FOR 2,000-CALORIE PLAN:

4 (4-ounce) salmon fillets

6 ounces trimmed asparagus

2 tablespoons lemon juice

2 cloves garlic, minced

1 teaspoon salt

1 teaspoon ground black pepper

Lemon slices, for garnish

1. Preheat the oven to 350°F. Line a rimmed baking sheet with parchment paper.

2. Arrange the salmon fillets, skin side down, on one side of the prepared baking.sheet. Dry the asparagus and arrange it on the other side of the baking sheet in one layer. Drizzle the lemon juice and sprinkle the garlic, salt, and pepper over everything. Bake until the salmon is opaque on the inside and the asparagus is tender, about 20 minutes.

3. Serve garnished with lemon slices.

1,500-CALORIE PLAN:

CALORIES:	PROTEIN:	CARBS:	FAT:
474	47g	4g	30g

2,000-CALORIE PLAN:

CALORIES:	PROTEIN:	CARBS:	FAT:
948	94g	8g	60g

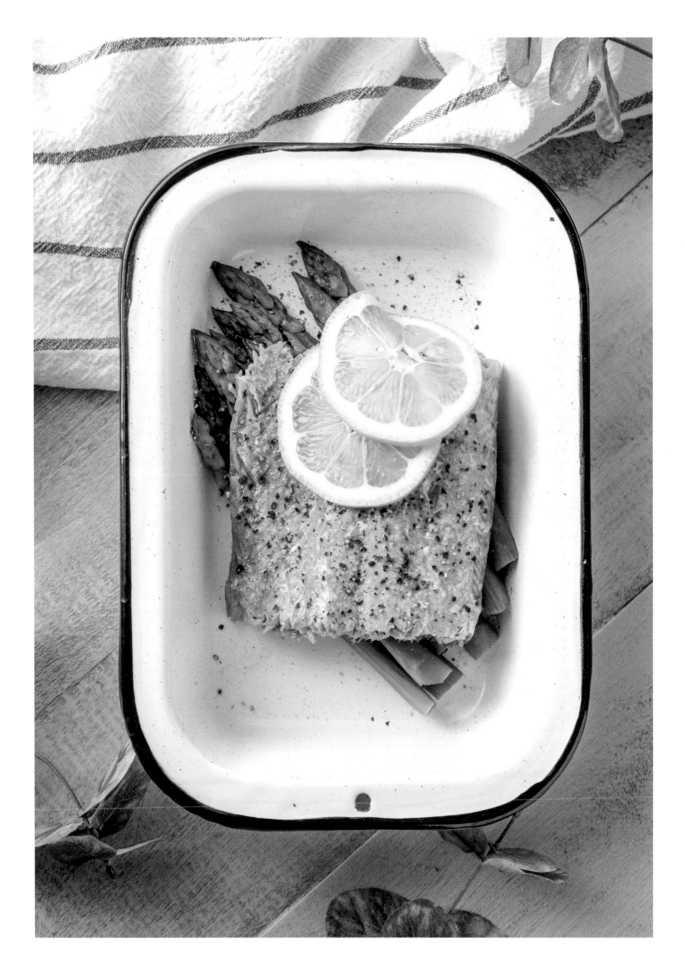

SWEDISH MEATBALLS & ARUGULA

MON TO THU

1 tablespoon finely chopped yellow or white onion

3 teaspoons extra-virgin olive oil, divided

2 tablespoons chopped fresh parsley

1 teaspoon finely chopped garlic

2 tablespoons blanched almond flour

1 ounce whey protein powder

1 large egg

1 teaspoon Worcestershire sauce

½ teaspoon ground allspice

¼ teaspoon ground nutmeg

½ teaspoon salt

½ teaspoon ground black pepper

3 ounces lean ground beef

1½ ounces lean ground pork

½ cup beef stock

¼ cup sour cream

¼ cup heavy cream

1 handful arugula

Finely chopped fresh parsley, for garnish

1. In a small skillet over medium heat, sauté the onion in 1½ teaspoons of the oil until translucent. Remove the pan from the heat and set aside.

2. In a small bowl, mix together the parsley, garlic, almond flour, whey protein powder, egg, Worcestershire sauce, allspice, nutmeg, salt, and pepper. Add the beef, pork, and sautéed onion and mix well. Using your hands, form the meat mixture into 1-inch balls.

3. In a medium skillet, heat the remaining 1½ teaspoons of olive oil over high heat. When the oil is hot, add the meatballs and cook until browned on the top and bottom.

4. Reduce the heat to medium. Keeping the skillet on the burner, use a pair of tongs to remove the meatballs from the skillet and set aside.

5. Add the beef stock, sour cream, and heavy cream to the medium skillet and stir well. Return the meatballs to the skillet and cook them in the sauce for another 20 minutes.

6. Put the arugula in a serving bowl and top with the meatballs and sauce. Garnish with parsley.

CALORIES:	PROTEIN:	CARBS:	FAT:
472	31g	6g	36g

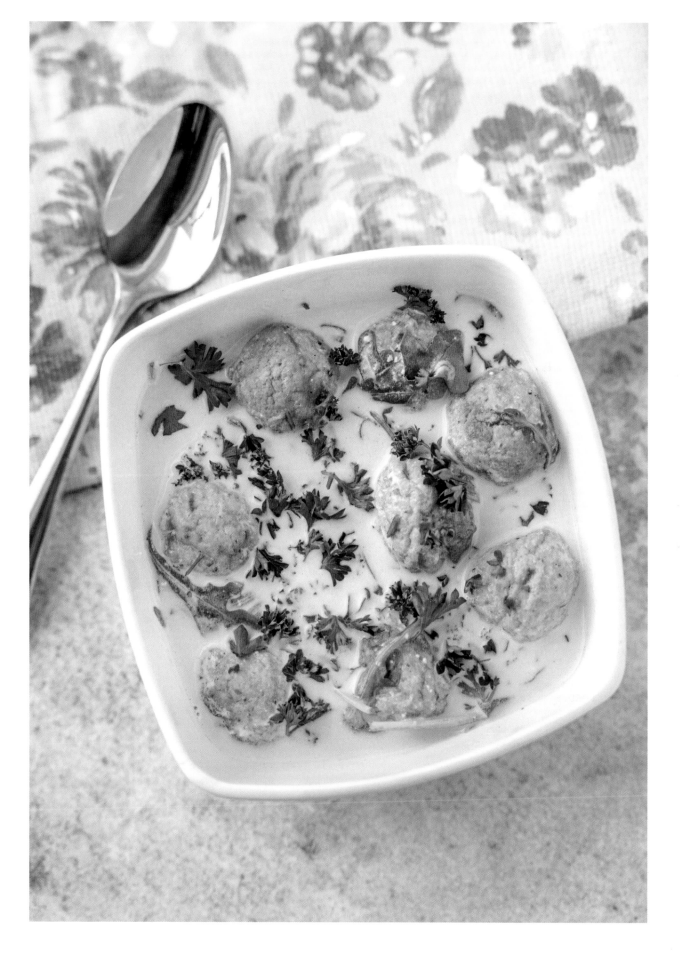

SWEET POTATO
EGG WHITE SCRAMBLE

FRI

9½ ounces peeled sweet potatoes, cut into 1-inch cubes

½ teaspoon salt

1 tablespoon extra-virgin olive oil

1 teaspoon ground cinnamon

7 large egg whites, or ¾ cup plus 2 tablespoons liquid egg whites

Ground black pepper

1 tablespoon chopped fresh herb of choice, such as chives, thyme, rosemary, oregano, or parsley

1. Put the sweet potatoes and salt in a medium saucepan. Cover with water and bring to a boil. Cook until just tender enough to pierce easily with the tip of a knife but still quite firm, 15 to 20 minutes. Drain well.

2. Heat the oil in a medium skillet over medium-high heat. Add the boiled sweet potatoes and cook until golden on all sides, about 3 minutes. Add the cinnamon and mix well. Transfer the sweet potatoes to a serving bowl.

3. In another bowl, lightly beat the egg whites with a fork until blended, then pour into the skillet. Stir with a rubber spatula until cooked through.

4. Top the sweet potatoes with the egg white scramble, season with pepper, and garnish with the chopped herb.

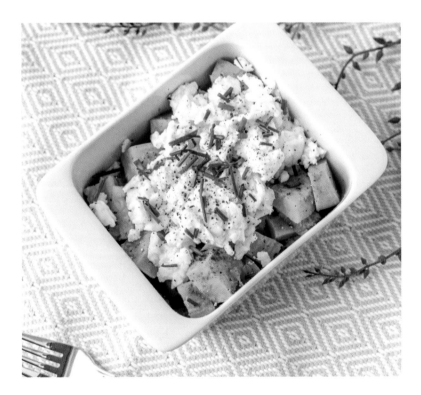

CALORIES:	PROTEIN:	CARBS:	FAT:
491	30g	59g	15g

BAKED BUTTERNUT SQUASH WITH ORANGE & RAISINS

5 cups peeled and cubed butternut squash

½ teaspoon salt

½ teaspoon ground black pepper

1 medium orange

3½ ounces plain low-fat yogurt, stirred

3 ounces raisins

1. Preheat the oven to 400°F. Line a rimmed baking sheet with parchment paper.

2. Put the squash in a bowl, sprinkle with the salt and pepper, and toss to mix well. Arrange the squash in a single layer on the prepared baking sheet and bake until golden and soft all the way through, about 40 minutes. Transfer to a serving plate and set aside to cool a bit.

3. Meanwhile, peel the orange and cut it into slices; add to the squash. Drizzle the yogurt over the squash and orange, top with the raisins, and serve.

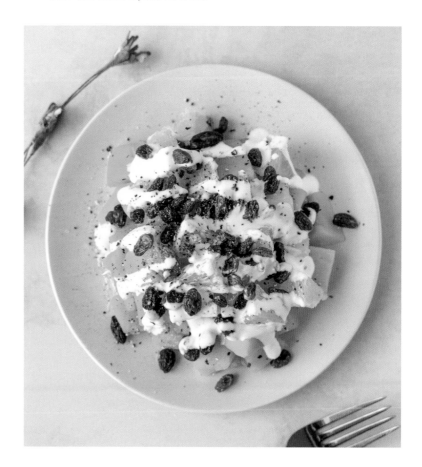

CALORIES:	PROTEIN:	CARBS:	FAT:
528	10g	113g	4g

FRI

AROMATIC RICE & CHICKEN

FOR 1,500-CALORIE PLAN:

½ cup basmati rice

2 star anise pods

2 cardamom pods

8 ounces boneless, skinless chicken breast

½ teaspoon salt

½ teaspoon ground black pepper

2 tablespoons chopped fresh cilantro

FOR 2,000-CALORIE PLAN:

1 cup basmati rice

4 star anise pods

4 cardamom pods

1 pound boneless, skinless chicken breasts, cut into ½-inch-thick cutlets

1 teaspoon salt

1 teaspoon ground black pepper

¼ cup chopped fresh cilantro

1. Cook the rice according to the package instructions, adding the star anise, cardamom, and salt to the pan when you add the rice. Once cooked, remove and discard the star anise and cardamom pods; fluff the rice with a fork.

2. Preheat a grill to medium-high heat. Grill the chicken until cooked through in the middle (check it with a fork), 10 to 15 minutes, turning it over halfway through. Sprinkle with the salt and pepper and remove from the heat.

3. Spoon the rice onto a serving plate and top with the chopped cilantro. Cut the chicken against the grain into ½-inch slices and arrange them on top of the rice.

1,500-CALORIE PLAN:			
CALORIES:	PROTEIN:	CARBS:	FAT:
492	38g	76g	4g

2,000-CALORIE PLAN:			
CALORIES:	PROTEIN:	CARBS:	FAT:
984	76g	152g	8g

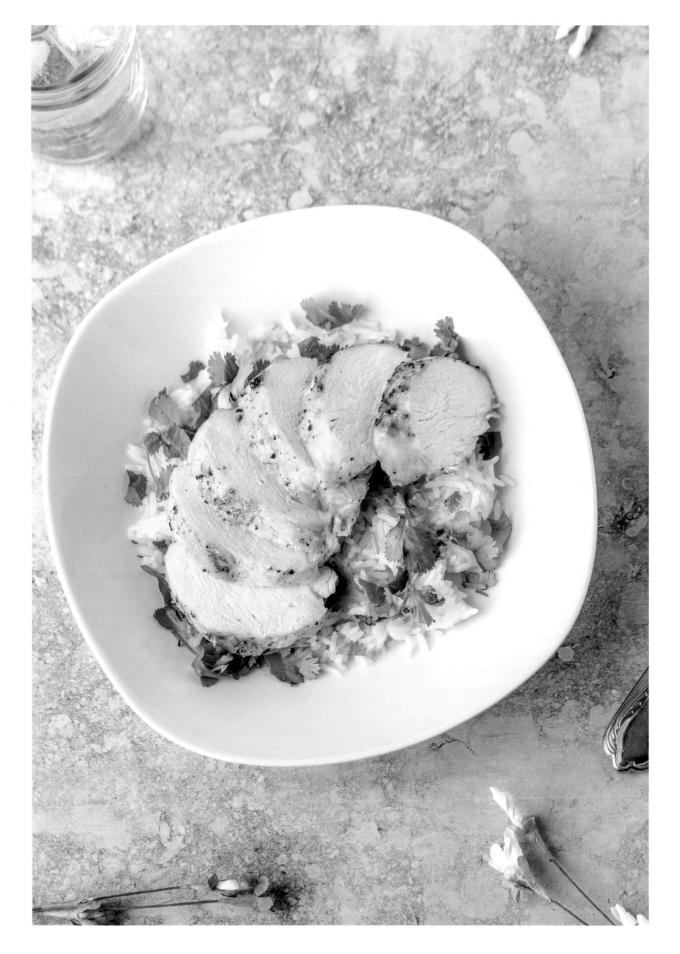

GARLIC RICE-STUFFED
PORTOBELLO MUSHROOMS

SAT

FOR 1,500-CALORIE PLAN:

½ cup basmati rice

1 teaspoon extra-virgin olive oil

4 (4-ounce) portobello mushrooms, stems removed

½ teaspoon salt

½ teaspoon ground black pepper

2 cloves garlic, minced

2 teaspoons fresh thyme leaves

Finely chopped fresh parsley, for garnish

FOR 2,000-CALORIE PLAN:

1 cup basmati rice

2 teaspoons extra-virgin olive oil

8 (4-ounce) portobello mushrooms, stems removed

1 teaspoon salt

1 teaspoon ground black pepper

4 cloves garlic, minced

4 teaspoons fresh thyme leaves

Finely chopped fresh parsley, for garnish

1. Cook the rice according to the package instructions. Season the cooking water with salt to taste.

2. While the rice is cooking, preheat a grill to medium heat. Coat the grates of the grill with the oil. Season the mushroom caps with the salt and pepper and grill until browned on both sides, 10 to 15 minutes. Transfer to a platter.

3. Fluff the rice with a fork and stir in the garlic and thyme. Top the mushroom caps evenly with the rice mixture. Garnish with parsley.

1,500-CALORIE PLAN:

CALORIES:	PROTEIN:	CARBS:	FAT:
527	22g	94g	7g

2,000-CALORIE PLAN:

CALORIES:	PROTEIN:	CARBS:	FAT:
1,054	44g	188g	14g

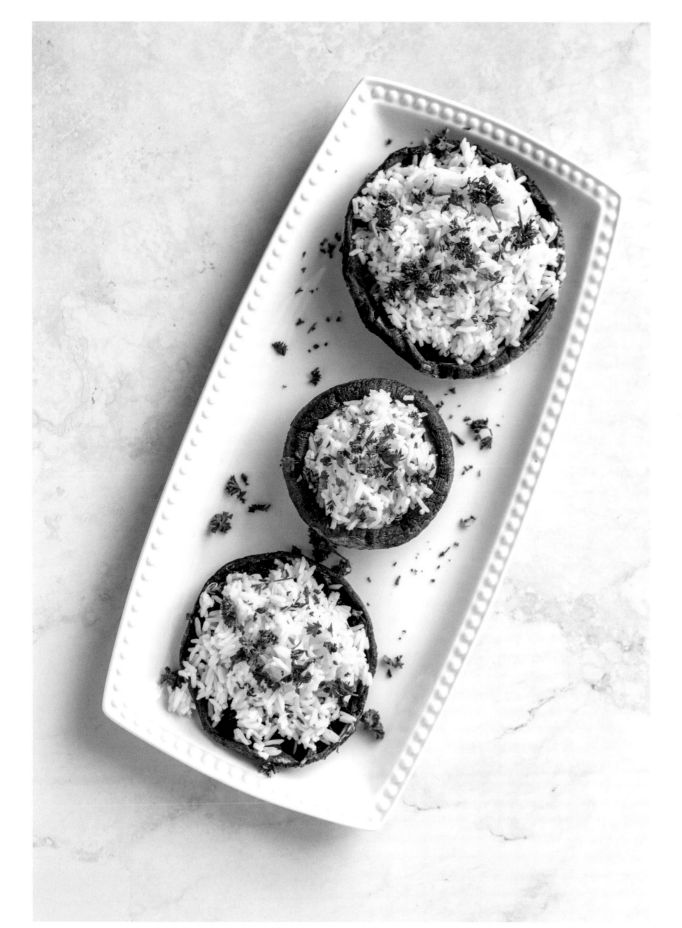

PULLED PORK TACOS WITH POTATOES

SAT

7 ounces waxy potatoes

1 medium tomato, finely chopped

1 tablespoon finely chopped onion

1 tablespoon lime juice

½ teaspoon salt

½ teaspoon ground black pepper

7½ ounces slow-cooked shredded pork (page 161)

3 large romaine lettuce leaves

Finely chopped fresh cilantro, for garnish

1. Cut the potatoes into small chunks and boil in a pot of salted water for 15 minutes, or until tender. Drain and set aside.

2. Make the salsa: In a small bowl, mix the tomato, onion, and lime juice, then season with the salt and pepper.

3. Place the lettuce leaves on a platter, spoon the pulled pork into the lettuce leaves, top with the salsa, and garnish with cilantro. Serve with a side of boiled potatoes (not shown).

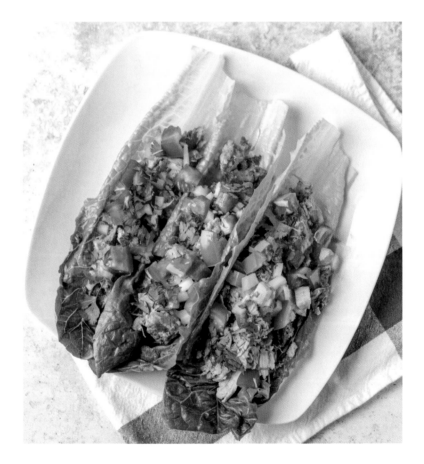

CALORIES:	PROTEIN:	CARBS:	FAT:
496	49g	39g	16g

BAKED TURKEY & APPLES

9 ounces boneless, skinless turkey breast, cut into ½-inch-thick cutlets

½ teaspoon salt

½ teaspoon ground black pepper

1 (8-ounce) Fuji apple

1 tablespoon lemon juice

1 tablespoon maple syrup

1 teaspoon extra-virgin olive oil

1 teaspoon ground cinnamon

1 sprig fresh thyme, finely chopped

1. Preheat the oven to 400°F. Line a rimmed baking sheet with parchment paper.

2. Place the turkey cutlets on the prepared baking sheet and season with the salt and pepper. Bake for 20 minutes.

3. Meanwhile, core and slice the apple. Arrange the slices on top of the turkey breast and bake for another 15 minutes, or until the turkey is cooked through. Remove from the oven.

4. Put the lemon juice, maple syrup, olive oil, cinnamon, and thyme in a small jar with a lid and shake to combine. Spoon the sauce over the turkey and apple slices and serve.

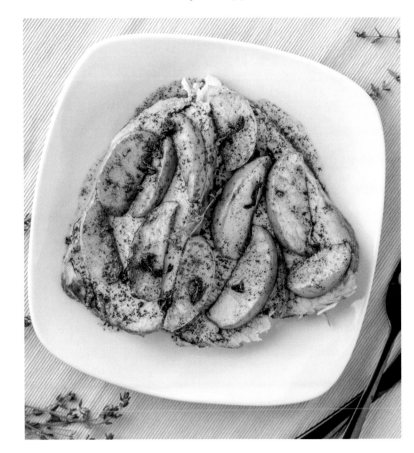

CALORIES:	PROTEIN:	CARBS:	FAT:
459	50g	49g	7g

ONE-WEEK CYCLICAL KETOGENIC DIET TRAINING PLAN

Monday	Keto-Specific Lower Body Training
Tuesday	Walking Recovery Day
Wednesday	Keto-Specific Upper Body Training
Thursday	Walking Recovery Day
Friday	Total Body Training*
Saturday	Total Body Training*
Sunday	Rest

These workouts are mandatory or you don't get your high-carb day. Do your Friday workout before your first carb-up. Your Saturday workout may be done at any time.

Please visit my YouTube channel for exercise demo videos: YouTube.com/coachtaragarrison.

UNDERSTANDING YOUR TRAINING PLAN

When you are in ketosis, your muscle glycogen (stored carbohydrate) levels are much lower, especially if you haven't been eating keto for very long. This impacts your performance during high-intensity exercise.

When you do all-out, intense exercise lasting from 30 seconds to about 2 minutes (think a 400-meter dash or 10 to 20 rep max lifts), your body runs off glycolysis, a process in which glycogen is broken down to make enough ATP (energy) to support the demand. So you perform better in these types of exercises when you have more glycogen stored in your body.

For this reason, the exercise intensity in this plan increases on Friday and Saturday when you are eating more carbs. If it works with your schedule, wait to have your first carbohydrate-rich meal until after Friday's workout. Although your exercise performance may not be at its peak, the demand will make your muscles like sponges for the incoming glucose after your workout. The longer you are adapted to keto, the more you will spare glycogen in your muscles, and the easier this workout will become over time on a cyclical ketogenic diet.

If you feel like you absolutely can't perform the workout on Friday, try adding 20 to 30 grams of a fast-acting carbohydrate like dextrose, glucose, or maltodextrin before your workout. You can get these in powdered form and add them to your pre-workout drink. I like a highly branched cyclic dextrin for this purpose because it is quickly digested and sends a steady stream of fuel to your muscles.

During aerobic exercise, generally when your heart rate is about 50 to 70 percent of your maximum, your body uses blood glucose and glycogen but also runs on fat. The longer you are keto, the better your body becomes at running on fat for fuel during aerobic exercise, and it will start sparing glycogen and favoring fat as a fuel source to support the activity. This heart rate can be achieved by walking briskly. For this reason, this plan includes two days of brisk walking while you are in ketosis to both train this system and assist in body fat loss. If you are a trained endurance athlete, you can run or bike on these days, but don't go at an all-out effort. Keep your heart rate at around 50 to 60 percent of your max; training toward the lower end of your aerobic range is ideal to make sure you stay in that fat-burning state and don't trickle into glycolysis.

For your weight training days while in ketosis, you do lower rep ranges and longer rest intervals because your body doesn't have as much glycogen to support higher rep ranges. Be sure to lift heavy so you get a stimulus from the training session; if you go low rep and low weight, you won't do much to stimulate muscle growth. Also, save your cardio for after your weight training so that the little bit of muscle glycogen you do have goes to support your lifts. This also puts your body in a low-glycogen state to encourage more fat oxidation during cardio.

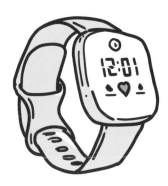

MONDAY: KETO-SPECIFIC LOWER BODY TRAINING

Warm up by walking on a treadmill for 5 to 10 minutes. Then complete the following sequence, resting for 60 to 75 seconds between sets.

1. Bodyweight Walking Lunges: 3 sets of 12/leg. Make sure your front heel is in contact with the floor before pushing up to standing. Keep your knee outside of your big toe to prevent injury.
   - Set 1: Body weight
   - Set 2: Hold medium-weight dumbbells at your sides
   - Set 3: Hold heavy dumbbells at your sides
2. Goblet Squats: 3 sets of 8. Distribute your weight in your entire foot, making sure you are bearing weight in your heels. Hold the dumbbell or kettlebell to your chest. Increase the weight with each set.
3. Romanian Deadlifts: 3 sets of 8. Use dumbbells or a barbell. Keep the weight close to your shins. Push your hips back and keep your weight in your heels.
4. Barbell Hip Thrusts: 3 sets of 8. Increase the weight with each set.
5. Leg Extensions: 3 sets of 8. Increase the weight with each set.
6. Lying Leg Curls: 3 sets of 8. Increase the weight with each set.
7. Barbell Glute Bridges from Floor: 3 sets of 8. Increase the weight with each set.
8. Seated or Standing Calf Raises: 3 sets of 8. Increase the weight with each set.

Finish with 20 minutes of cardio. You can walk briskly or use another cardio method of your choice at 50 to 60 percent of your max heart rate.

> NOTE: If you don't know your max heart rate, subtract your age from 180 to estimate it. Or go just hard enough that you work up a bit of a sweat while still being able to hold a conversation.

TUESDAY: WALKING RECOVERY DAY

Do 60 minutes of brisk walking or another cardio method of your choice at 50 to 60 percent of your max heart rate, or go just hard enough that you work up a bit of a sweat while still being able to hold a conversation.

WEDNESDAY: KETO-SPECIFIC UPPER BODY TRAINING

Warm up by walking on a treadmill for 5 to 10 minutes. Then complete the following sequence, resting for 60 to 75 seconds between sets and increasing the weight with each set.

1. Seated Dumbbell Overhead Presses: 3 sets of 8.
2. Dumbbell Biceps Curls: 3 sets of 8.
3. Cable Rope Triceps Extensions: 3 sets of 8.
4. Dumbbell Lateral Raises: 3 sets of 8.
5. Dumbbell Biceps Hammer Curls: 3 sets of 8.
6. Dumbbell Skull Crushers: 3 sets of 8.
7. Dumbbell Bench Presses: 3 sets of 8.
8. Bent-Over Rows: 3 sets of 16 (8/arm).

Finish with 20 minutes of cardio. Walk briskly or do another cardio method of your choice at 50 to 60 percent of your max heart rate.

THURSDAY: WALKING RECOVERY DAY

Do 60 minutes of brisk walking or another cardio method of your choice at 50 to 60 percent of your max heart rate.

FRIDAY: TOTAL BODY TRAINING

Warm up by walking on a treadmill for 5 to 10 minutes.

Today's workout includes giant sets, in which you do all the exercises consecutively without rest and then rest at the end of the set, which is appropriate if you work out later in the day or after you eat carbs. However, if you train in the morning before you carb up, give yourself 60 seconds of rest between exercises.

GIANT SET 1: LEGS, CHEST, AND BACK

Do one set of each exercise, moving immediately to the next exercise in the list. Rest for 2 minutes before restarting the giant set with the first exercise. Complete 3 giant sets.

1. **24 Step-Ups (12/leg):** Hold dumbbells at your sides. Make sure your full foot, including your heel, makes contact with the platform. Increase the weight with each set.

2. **12 Push-Ups:** You may elevate your hands on a box if you can't do flat push-ups. Place plates on your back or wear a weighted vest if unweighted push-ups are too easy for you.

3. **12 Romanian Deadlifts or Hex Bar Deadlifts:** Increase the weight with each set.

4. **12 Seated Cable Rows or Chest-Supported Dumbbell Rows:** Increase the weight with each set.

GIANT SET 2: SHOULDERS, BICEPS, AND TRICEPS

Do one set of each exercise, moving immediately to the next exercise in the list. Rest for 2 minutes before restarting the giant set with the first exercise. Complete 3 giant sets.

1. **12 Dumbbell Front Raises for shoulders**

2. **12 Seated Dumbbell Biceps Curls**

3. **12 Dumbbell Lateral Raises for shoulders**

4. **12 Dumbbell Skull Crushers**

5. **12 Bent-Over Dumbbell Rows for rear delts**

Finish with 20 minutes of cardio. Walk briskly or do another cardio method of your choice at 50 to 60 percent of your max heart rate.

SATURDAY: TOTAL BODY TRAINING

Today you will do supersets that have one resistance training exercise followed by one plyometric exercise. The extra carbs will aid your athletic performance and allow you to be more explosive, so the plan takes advantage of that to both increase your athleticism and make sure you are using the carbs you are eating intelligently.

Take as little rest as possible between exercises in a superset. In other words, immediately follow your weightlifting movement with your plyometric movement. Then rest between supersets as prescribed.

Warm up by walking on a treadmill for 5 to 10 minutes.

LOWER BODY SUPERSET

Do the superset three times, resting for 60 seconds between sets.

1. 20 Weighted Walking Lunges (10/leg): Hold dumbbells at your sides and increase the weight with each set.
2. 20 Banded Lateral Side Hops (10 to each side)

UPPER BODY SUPERSET

Do the superset three times, resting for 60 seconds between sets.

1. 15 Lat Pulldowns
2. 15 Medicine Ball Slams

LOWER BODY SUPERSET

Do the superset three times, resting for 60 seconds between sets.

1. 15 Double Kettlebell Rack Hold Squats (or Goblet Squats)
2. 15 Jumping Squats

UPPER BODY SUPERSET

Do the superset three times, resting for 60 seconds between sets.

1. 15 Dumbbell Bench Presses
2. 15 Medicine Ball Chest Passes (against a wall)

TOTAL BODY SUPERSET FINISHER

Do the superset three times, resting for 60 seconds between sets.

1. 40 Kettlebell Snatches (20/arm)
2. 5 Man Makers

Finish with 20 minutes of cardio speed intervals using the cardio method of your choice. Warm up for 5 minutes. Then go all-out for 30 seconds, followed by 2 minutes at a normal pace. Repeat for 15 minutes.

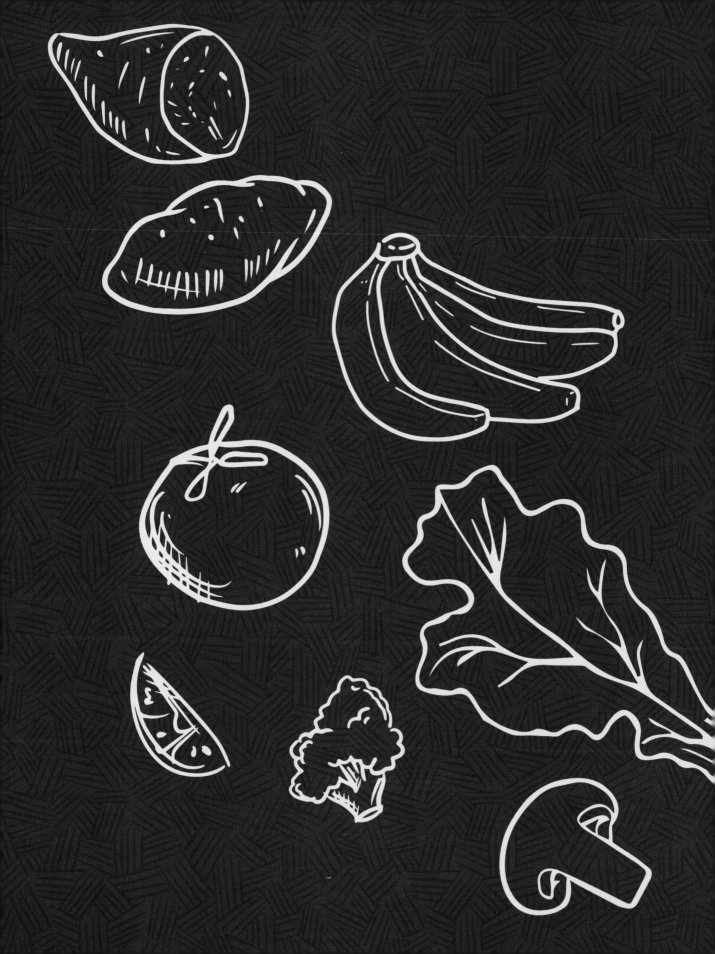

FOUR-WEEK BRING-BACK-THE-CARBS PLAN

FOUR-WEEK BRING-BACK-THE-CARBS MEAL PLAN

You will gradually increase your carbohydrate intake over this four-week plan. This gives your digestive tract time to get used to the incremental increase in fiber and gives your body time to increase the production of amylase, the enzyme that breaks down carbs. This way, your body won't get slammed with a ton of carbs all at once when it's not used to them and have a hard time digesting those carbs.

While I encourage you to add vegetables to your diet, if you go overboard and add a lot of veggies at once, you will likely experience some uncomfortable gas and bloating. Slow, steady increases are the better way to go.

If you have an autoimmune disease or food sensitivities, please swap out any foods on this plan to which you have a sensitivity for something you can have. Also, keep an eye out for any foods that cause you extreme bloating, gas, nausea, stomach pain, heartburn, diarrhea, headaches, or acne. You may be sensitive to these foods without realizing it, and you will want to swap them out for foods that your body tolerates well.

Make sure you also increase your water intake to help indigestible fiber pass through your intestines.

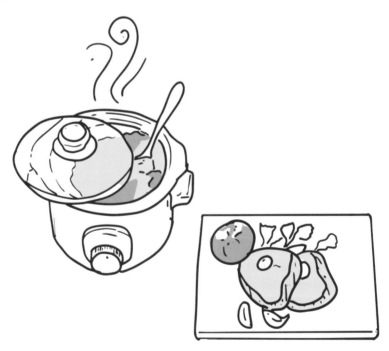

HOW TO CONFIGURE YOUR CALORIES:

- **For fat loss:** Multiply your body weight in pounds by 10. If you are not losing fat on this number of calories, or if the restriction is way too intense and you're absolutely starving, move your calorie intake up or down a little until you find your sweet spot.

- **For maintenance:** Multiply your body weight in pounds by 13 or 14. You may have to play with your calorie intake a little, moving it up or down until you find your sweet spot.

- **For mass gain:** Multiply your body weight in pounds by 15 or 16. You may have to play with your calorie intake a little, moving it up or down until you find your sweet spot.

PLEASE NOTE:

- The 1,500-Calorie Plan is designed for fat loss and muscle growth for a 150-pound person. The 2,000-Calorie Plan is designed for fat loss and muscle growth for a 200-pound person. These are merely examples. Use the formulas I have provided to find your appropriate caloric intake.
- If you are following the 2,000-Calorie Plan, you will simply eat a double portion of one meal every day, as marked by asterisks.
- I recommend that you batch-cook the meats for the week in a slow cooker. On average, raw meat loses 25 percent of its weight once cooked.
- Almost all of the recipes make one serving. Only two recipes make more than that, and it's noted in those recipes.

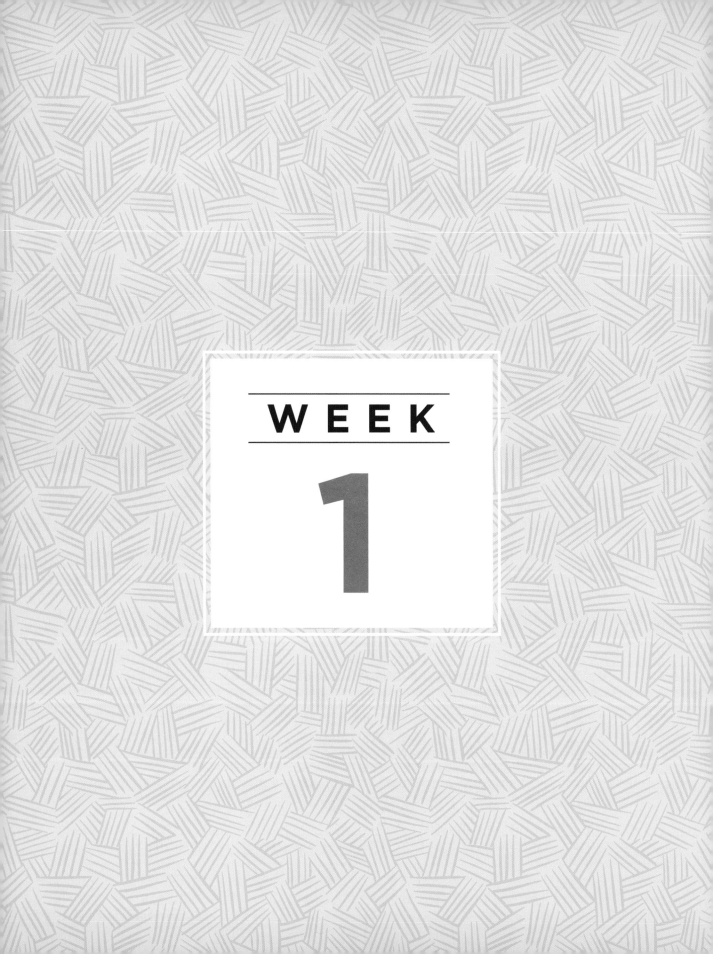

WEEK

1

		1,500-CALORIE PLAN		2,000-CALORIE PLAN	
MONDAY to WEDNESDAY	**Breakfast:** Chocolate Almond Butter Protein Shake* (page 192) **Lunch:** Crispy-Skin Salmon with Cauliflower Rice (page 194) **Dinner:** Chicken & Brussels Sprouts with Toasted Pine Nuts (page 196)	Calories:	**1,581**	Calories:	**2,100**
		Protein:	**167g**	Protein:	**226g**
		Carbs:	**73g**	Carbs:	**110g**
		Fat:	**69g**	Fat:	**84g**
THURSDAY to SATURDAY	**Breakfast:** Bacon Egg Muffins with Sour Cream* (page 198) **Lunch:** High-Protein Niçoise Salad (page 200) **Dinner:** Shredded Beef with Spicy Lime Quinoa (page 202)	Calories:	**1,517**	Calories:	**1,981**
		Protein:	**141g**	Protein:	**180g**
		Carbs:	**83g**	Carbs:	**97g**
		Fat:	**69g**	Fat:	**97g**
SUNDAY	**Breakfast:** Raspberry Protein Pancake* (page 204) **Lunch:** Oregano Chicken with Wilted Greens (page 206) **Dinner:** Potato Sandwiches with Creamy Radish Spread (page 208)	Calories:	**1,599**	Calories:	**2,036**
		Protein:	**157g**	Protein:	**179g**
		Carbs:	**92g**	Carbs:	**114g**
		Fat:	**67g**	Fat:	**96g**

If you are following the 2,000-Calorie Plan, you will eat a double portion of this meal.

Instructions for slow-cooking the chicken for the week ahead:

Place 1¾ pounds boneless, skinless chicken breasts in a slow cooker with 2 teaspoons salt, 2 teaspoons ground black pepper, 1 clove garlic, and 1 bay leaf. Cook on low for 4 hours. Take the meat out of the slow cooker and pull it apart using two forks.

Instructions for slow-cooking the beef for the week ahead:

Place 17 ounces boneless beef shank in a slow cooker with 2 teaspoons salt, 2 teaspoons ground black pepper, 1 clove garlic, and 1 bay leaf. Cook on low for 4 hours. Take the meat out of the slow cooker and pull it apart using two forks.

WEEK 1 SHOPPING LIST

*Additional quantities for the 2,000-Calorie Plan are marked with an asterisk.

MEAT, EGGS & DAIRY:

Bacon, 3 slices

Boneless beef shank, 17 ounces

Boneless, skinless chicken breasts, 2¼ pounds

Cottage cheese, 14 ounces

Egg whites, 12 large, or 1½ cups liquid egg whites (*add 12 large egg whites or 1½ cups liquid egg whites)

Eggs, 15 large (*add 9)

Grass-fed unsalted butter, 1 stick

Greek yogurt, plain full-fat, 1½ ounces

Skin-on salmon fillets, 1½ pounds

Sour cream, 1 small container

FRESH PRODUCE:

Bananas, 3 medium (*add 3)

Basil, 1 bunch

Brussels sprouts, 12 ounces

Cauliflower, 1 medium head

Chives, 1 bunch

Dill, 1 bunch

Fennel, 1 bulb

Garlic, 3 cloves

Green beans, 4½ ounces

Kale, 1 bunch

Lemons, 4

Limes, 3

Orange, 1 medium

Oregano, 1 bunch

Radishes, 5 medium

Raspberries, 1 cup

Red onion, 1 small

Red potatoes, small, 7½ ounces

Romaine lettuce, 1 head

Russet potato, 1 medium (about 5 ounces)

Thyme, 1 bunch

Yellow or white onion, 1

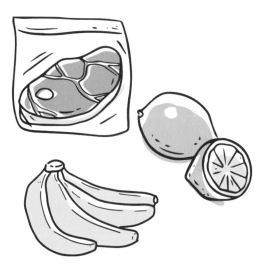

PANTRY & FREEZER ITEMS:

Almond butter, 3 tablespoons
(*add 3 tablespoons)

Almond, coconut, or cashew milk,
unsweetened, 1½ cups (*add 1½ cups)

Blanched almond flour, ⅓ cup

Chunk light tuna in water, 3 (5-ounce)
cans

Coconut milk, canned unsweetened
full-fat, 1 cup

Extra-virgin olive oil, 8¼ ounces
(*add ¾ ounce)

Honey, 3 tablespoons

Peas, frozen or canned, 12 ounces (*add
12 ounces)

Pine nuts, 7 teaspoons

Powdered monkfruit sweetener,
2 tablespoons

Prepared yellow mustard, 1½ teaspoons

Quinoa, 7 ounces

Sugar-free maple syrup, 3 tablespoons
(optional, for the pancake)

Vanilla extract, 1½ teaspoons (*add
1½ teaspoons)

Whey protein powder, 8 ounces
(*add 6 ounces)

SPICES & SEEDS:

Bay leaves

Black peppercorns

Cayenne pepper

Dried oregano leaves

Ground cinnamon

Salt

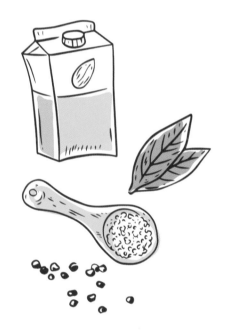

CHOCOLATE ALMOND BUTTER
PROTEIN SHAKE

MON TO WED

FOR 1,500-CALORIE PLAN:

⅔ cup ice cubes

½ cup unsweetened almond, coconut, or cashew milk

½ teaspoon vanilla extract

2 ounces whey protein powder

1 medium banana

1 tablespoon almond butter

Pinch of salt

FOR 2,000-CALORIE PLAN:

1⅓ cups ice cubes

1 cup unsweetened almond, coconut, or cashew milk

1 teaspoon vanilla extract

4 ounces whey protein powder

2 medium bananas

2 tablespoons almond butter

Pinch of salt

Whiz all the ingredients in a blender. Add water if needed to achieve the desired consistency. Pour into a tall glass and serve immediately.

1,500-CALORIE PLAN:			
CALORIES:	PROTEIN:	CARBS:	FAT:
519	59g	37g	15g

2,000-CALORIE PLAN:			
CALORIES:	PROTEIN:	CARBS:	FAT:
1038	118g	74g	30g

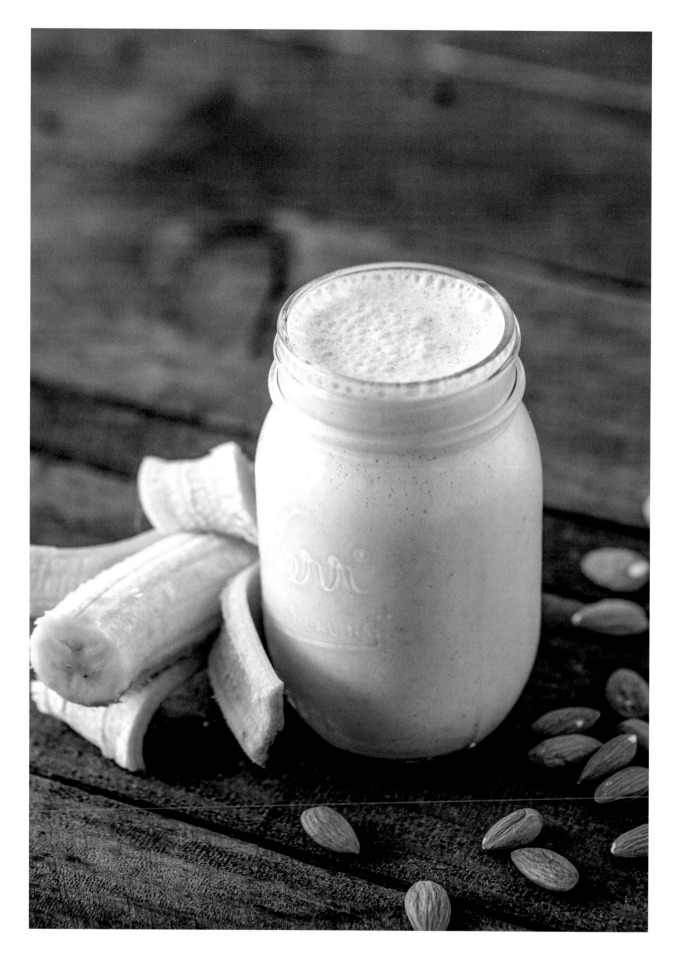

CRISPY-SKIN SALMON WITH CAULIFLOWER RICE

MON TO WED

2 teaspoons extra-virgin olive oil, divided

1 (7-ounce) skin-on salmon fillet

½ teaspoon salt, divided

½ teaspoon ground black pepper, divided

1 cup roughly chopped cauliflower

Juice of ½ lemon (optional)

Lemon slices, for garnish

Fresh parsley sprigs, for garnish

1. Preheat a medium skillet over medium-high heat. When hot, add 1 teaspoon of the oil. Place the salmon skin side down in the pan and cook for a few minutes to crisp the skin. Season with ¼ teaspoon each of the salt and pepper. Carefully flip the fillet, cover the skillet with a lid, reduce the heat to medium-low, and cook until the fish flakes easily with a fork, about 5 minutes.

2. Meanwhile, whiz the cauliflower in a blender until it is in pieces the size of grains of rice.

3. Transfer the salmon to a serving plate, leaving the burner on and keeping the salmon juices in the skillet. Add the remaining 1 teaspoon of oil to the skillet, turn the heat up to high, and cook the riced cauliflower until slightly golden, about 5 minutes. Stir in the remaining ¼ teaspoon each of the salt and pepper.

4. Drizzle the lemon juice over the salmon, if using. Garnish with lemon slices and parsley sprigs and serve with the cauliflower rice.

CALORIES:	PROTEIN:	CARBS:	FAT:
511	42g	7g	35g

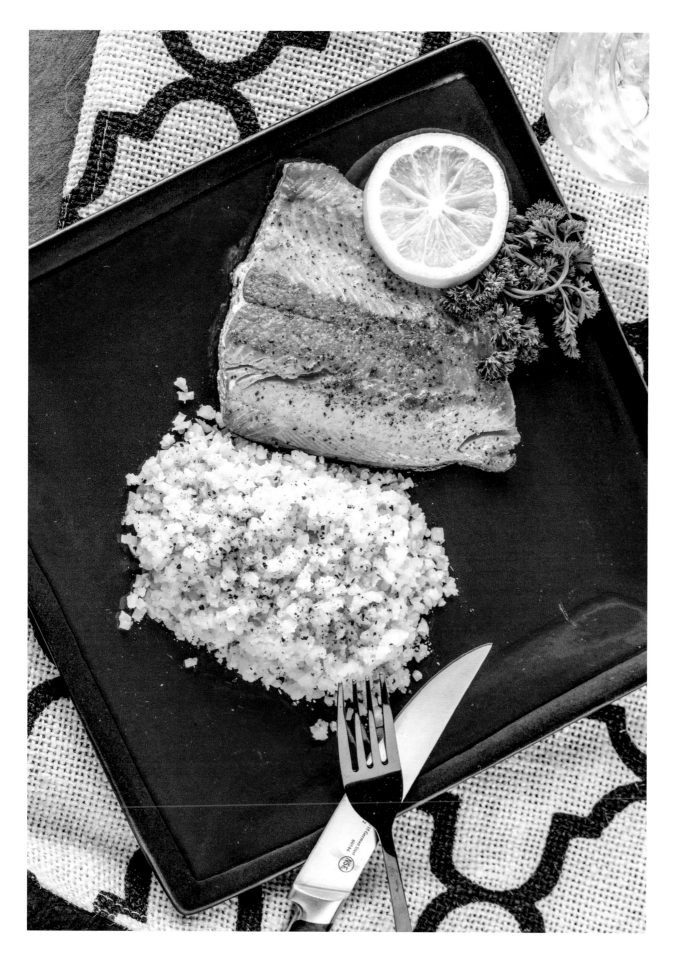

CHICKEN & BRUSSELS SPROUTS WITH
TOASTED PINE NUTS

2¼ teaspoons pine nuts

1 tablespoon extra-virgin olive oil

4 ounces Brussels sprouts, halved

½ teaspoon salt

7 ounces slow-cooked boneless, skinless chicken breast (page 189), shredded

1 tablespoon honey

1. Toast the pine nuts in a small skillet over medium heat, stirring frequently, until golden, about 2 minutes. Transfer to a plate to cool.

2. Wipe the skillet clean, add the oil, Brussels sprouts, and salt, and place over medium-high heat. Cook, stirring occasionally, until the sprouts are golden, about 4 minutes. Stir in the shredded chicken and heat through.

3. Transfer to a serving plate. Serve immediately drizzled with the honey and topped with the toasted pine nuts.

CALORIES:	PROTEIN:	CARBS:	FAT:
551	66g	29g	19g

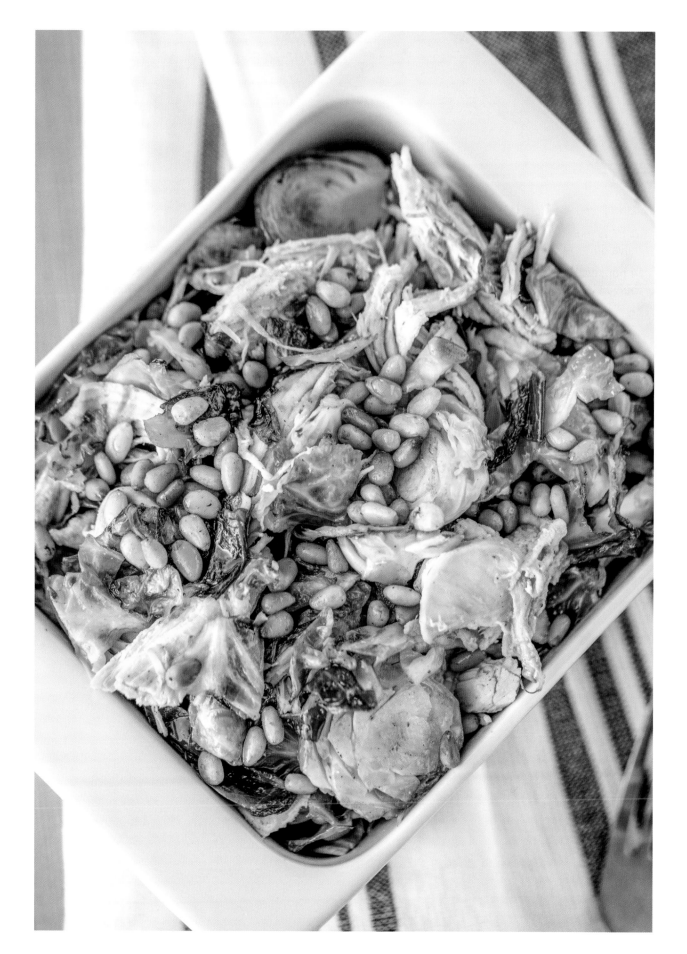

BACON EGG MUFFINS WITH SOUR CREAM

THU
TO
SAT

MAKES *12 muffins*

1,500-CALORIE PLAN: *Have 6 muffins*

2,000-CALORIE PLAN: *Have 12 muffins*

1 tablespoon extra-virgin olive oil, for the pan

6 large eggs

8 large egg whites, or 1 cup liquid egg whites

½ teaspoon salt

½ teaspoon ground black pepper

1 cup frozen or canned peas, drained

1 tablespoon chopped fresh chives

2 slices bacon, finely chopped

¼ cup sour cream, for serving

Thinly sliced scallions, for garnish

1. Preheat the oven to 375°F. Grease a standard-size 12-cup muffin tin with the oil.

2. Whiz the eggs, egg whites, salt, and pepper in a blender until homogeneous. Stir in the peas, chives, and bacon.

3. Divide the egg mixture evenly among the cups of the prepared muffin tin. Bake until the tops are golden brown and slightly firm to the touch, about 20 minutes. Set aside to cool.

4. Top each muffin with 1 teaspoon of sour cream. Garnish with scallions.

1,500-CALORIE PLAN:

CALORIES:	PROTEIN:	CARBS:	FAT:
464	39g	14g	28g

2,000-CALORIE PLAN:

CALORIES:	PROTEIN:	CARBS:	FAT:
928	78g	28g	56g

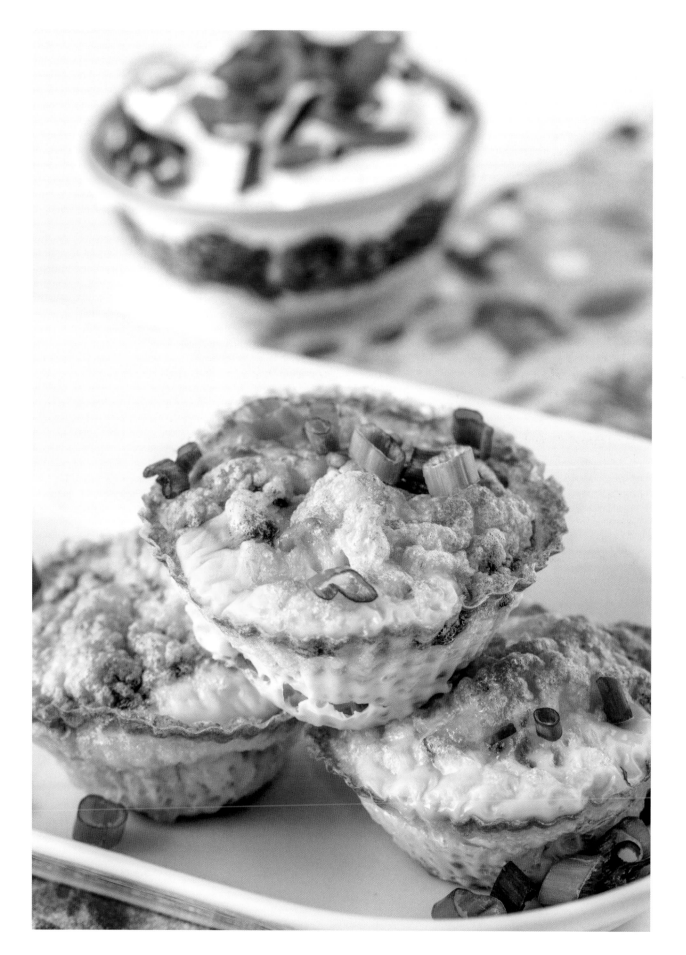

LUNCH

HIGH-PROTEIN
NIÇOISE SALAD

SALAD:

1 small new red potato

Salt

4 green beans

1 large egg

2 leaves romaine lettuce, torn into bite-sized pieces

⅛ small red onion, diced

1 (5-ounce) can chunk light tuna in water, well drained

VINAIGRETTE:

(Makes enough for 3 salads)

¼ cup plus 2 tablespoons lemon juice

3 tablespoons extra-virgin olive oil

3 tablespoons finely chopped red onions

1½ tablespoons finely chopped fresh basil

1½ tablespoons finely chopped fresh oregano

1½ tablespoons finely chopped fresh thyme

1½ teaspoons prepared yellow mustard

Salt, to taste

1. Place the potato in a small saucepan and cover with water. Add a generous amount of salt. Bring to a boil, then lower the heat to maintain a simmer. Cook until the potato is fork-tender, 10 to 12 minutes, then drain.

2. In the meantime, boil the green beans in another small saucepan for a few minutes, until bright green and just tender. Transfer to a bowl with ice-cold water to shock them and stop the cooking process, then drain.

3. Hard-boil the egg in another small saucepan for 10 minutes. Rinse the egg immediately with cold water to make it easier to peel.

4. While the potato is still warm, cut it into bite-sized pieces. Peel and quarter the egg.

5. Make the vinaigrette: Put all the ingredients in a jar, screw the lid on tightly, and shake vigorously.

6. Put the potato, green beans, and onions in a small bowl and toss with one-third of the vinaigrette. (Store the leftover vinaigrette in the refrigerator for use over the next two days.) Place the lettuce on a plate and arrange the potato mixture, egg, and tuna on top.

CALORIES:	PROTEIN:	CARBS:	FAT:
537	48g	21g	29g

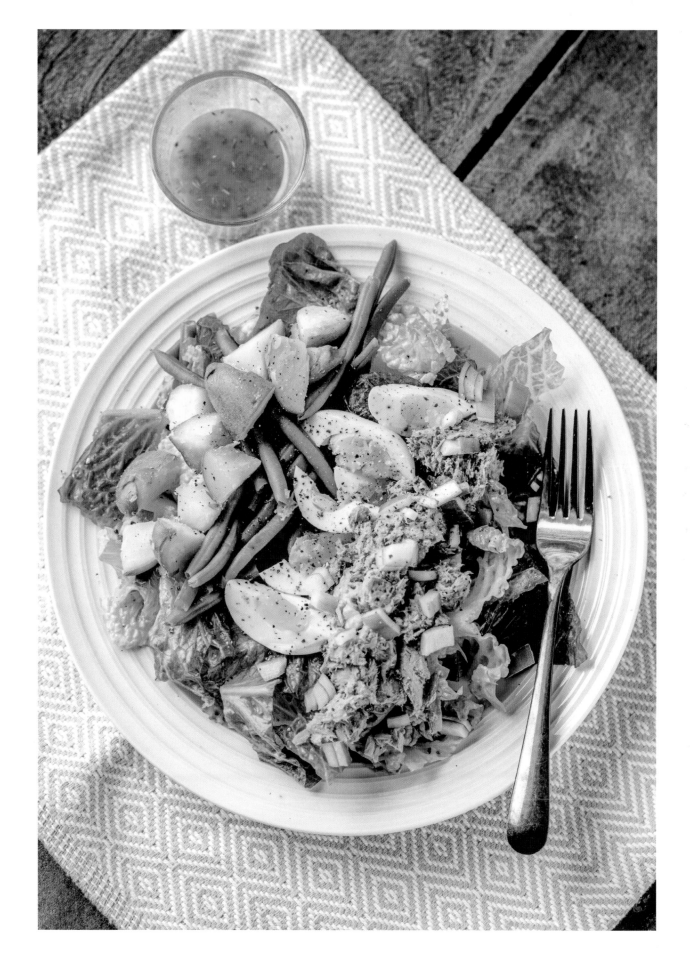

SHREDDED BEEF
WITH SPICY LIME
QUINOA

THU
TO
SAT

2⅓ ounces quinoa

⅓ medium orange, diced

1 tablespoon lime juice

½ teaspoon cayenne pepper

4½ ounces slow-cooked beef shank (page 189), warmed

1½ tablespoons thinly sliced scallions, for garnish

Cook the quinoa according to the package instructions. Drain well and place in a medium bowl. Add the diced orange, lime juice, and cayenne pepper and mix well. Serve the quinoa next to the beef and garnish with the scallions.

CALORIES:	PROTEIN:	CARBS:	FAT:
516	54g	48g	12g

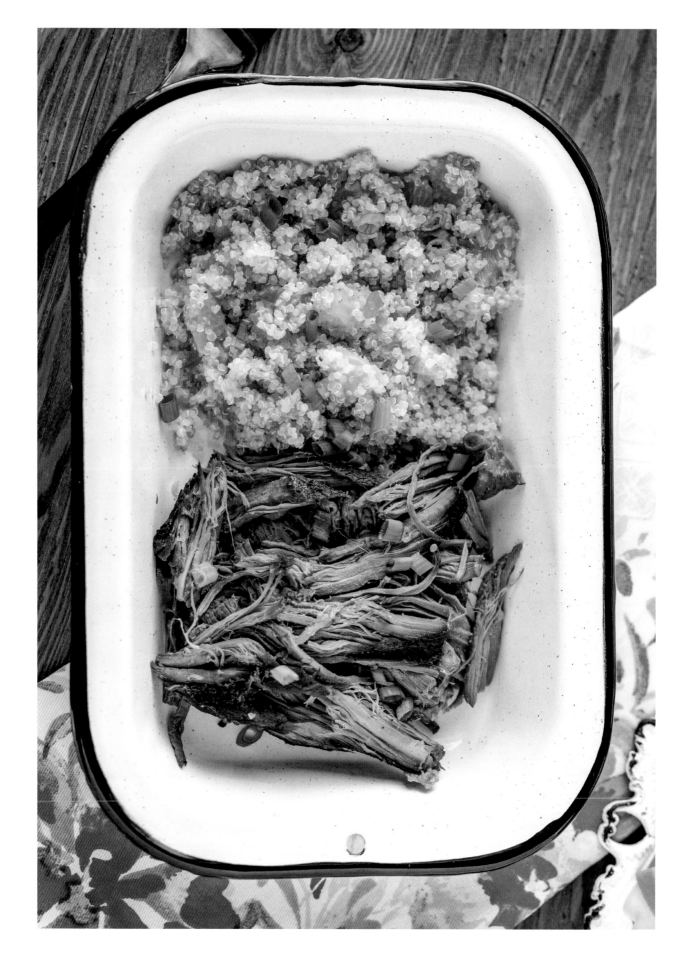

SUN

RASPBERRY
PROTEIN PANCAKE

MAKES *2 or 4 servings, depending on plan*

1,500-CALORIE PLAN: *Have 1 piece of 4*

2,000-CALORIE PLAN: *Have 2 pieces of 4*

3 large eggs

1 cup unsweetened full-fat canned coconut milk

⅓ cup blanched almond flour

2 ounces whey protein powder

½ teaspoon ground cinnamon

¼ teaspoon salt

¼ cup (½ stick) unsalted butter

1 cup raspberries

2 tablespoons powdered monkfruit sweetener, plus extra for sprinkling if desired

¼ cup maple syrup or honey, for drizzling

1. Preheat the oven to 400°F.

2. In a bowl, whisk together the eggs, coconut milk, almond flour, whey protein, cinnamon, and salt; set aside.

3. Heat the butter in an ovenproof 12-inch skillet (see note) over medium heat. Add the raspberries and monkfruit sweetener and stir until heated through. Remove the skillet from the heat and pour the batter into it, swirling to coat the surface.

4. Bake until the pancake is firm in the center, about 20 minutes. Let cool a bit before cutting into quarters and serving warm. Drizzle each portion with 1 tablespoon of maple syrup or honey and sprinkle with sweetener, if desired.

Note: If you don't have an ovenproof skillet, you can bake the pancake in a 13 by 9-inch baking dish, as shown.

1,500-CALORIE PLAN:			
CALORIES:	PROTEIN:	CARBS:	FAT:
437	22g	20g	29g

2,000-CALORIE PLAN:			
CALORIES:	PROTEIN:	CARBS:	FAT:
874	44g	40g	58g

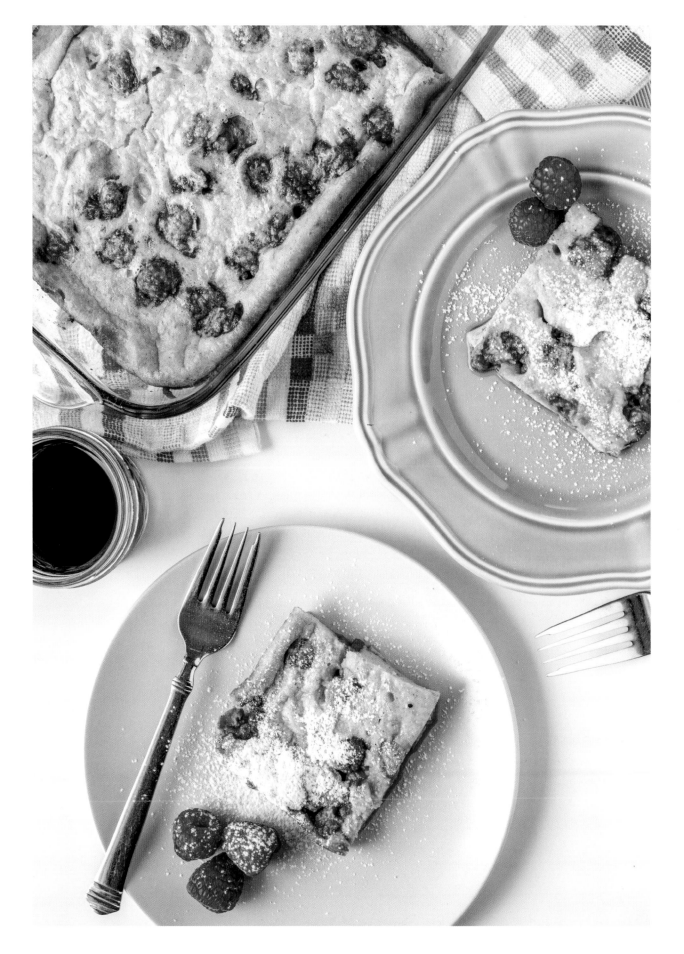

OREGANO CHICKEN
WITH WILTED GREENS

SUN

9 ounces boneless, skinless chicken breasts, cut against the grain into 1-inch-thick slices

½ teaspoon salt

½ teaspoon ground black pepper

2 tablespoons dried oregano leaves

1 tablespoon extra-virgin olive oil

¼ cup chopped yellow or white onions

1 bulb fennel, trimmed, cored, and diced

1½ cups destemmed and chopped kale

1. Preheat a grill to high heat, or preheat the oven to 375°F.

2. Rub the chicken breast slices with the salt, pepper, and oregano. Grill on both sides, 5 minutes per side, or bake until cooked through, about 25 minutes.

3. While the chicken is cooking, heat the oil in a medium skillet over medium-high heat. Add the onions and fennel and sauté until softened, about 3 minutes. Stir in the kale. Season with salt to taste and cook, stirring often, until the kale is wilted, about 2 more minutes.

4. Arrange the chicken on top of the vegetables.

CALORIES:	PROTEIN:	CARBS:	FAT:
609	85g	29g	17g

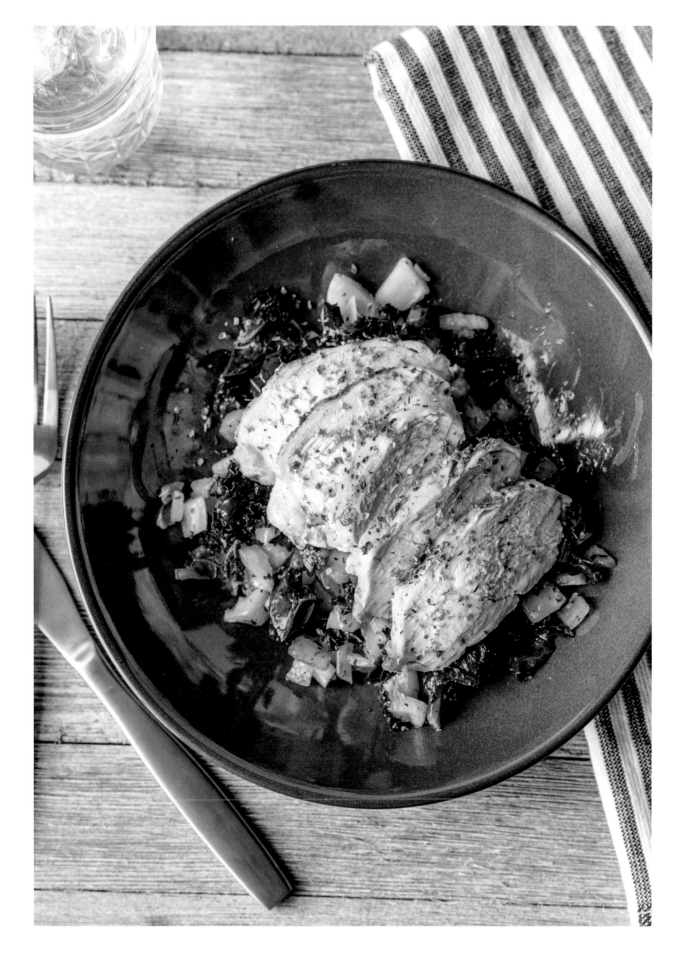

POTATO SANDWICHES
WITH CREAMY
RADISH SPREAD

SUN

1 medium russet potato
(about 5 ounces)

2 tablespoons extra-virgin
olive oil

Salt

RADISH SPREAD:

5 medium radishes

2 tablespoons fresh dill

1¾ cups full-fat cottage
cheese

3 tablespoons plain full-fat
Greek yogurt

Salt

1. Preheat the oven to 375°F. Line a rimmed baking sheet with parchment paper.

2. Peel the potato, then rinse and dry it. Place the potato on its side on a cutting board and carefully cut it lengthwise into an even number of slices, about ½ inch thick. Lay the potato slices on the prepared baking sheet. Drizzle with the oil and sprinkle with salt. Bake until the slices are golden brown and crispy on top, about 40 minutes.

3. While the potato is baking, dice the radishes and finely chop the dill. In a bowl, whisk together the cottage cheese and yogurt, then mix in the radishes and dill. Season with salt to taste.

4. Top half of the warm potato slices with the radish spread, then top with the other half of the potato slices to make "sandwiches."

CALORIES:	PROTEIN:	CARBS:	FAT:
553	50g	41g	21g

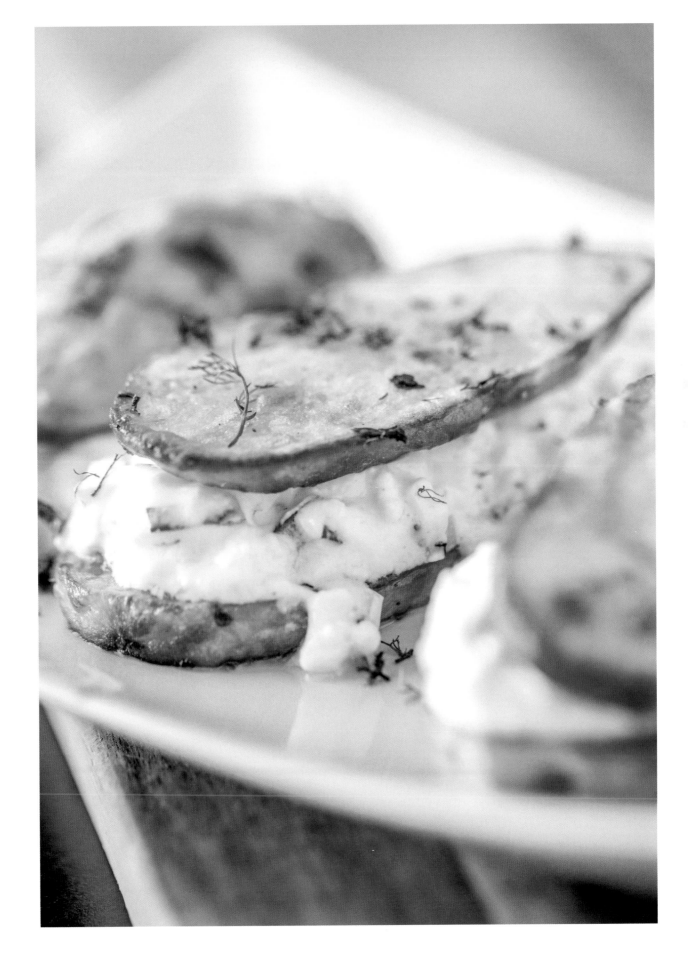

WEEK

2

		1,500-CALORIE PLAN		2,000-CALORIE PLAN	
MONDAY to WEDNESDAY	**Breakfast:** Mocha Protein Shake* (page 214) **Lunch:** Rosemary Beef & "Cheesy" Kale Salad (page 215) **Dinner:** Tart Apple Chicken Salad (page 216)	Calories:	1,580	Calories:	2,113
		Protein:	167g	Protein:	221g
		Carbs:	102g	Carbs:	143g
		Fat:	56g	Fat:	73g
THURSDAY to SATURDAY	**Breakfast:** Mushroom, Onion & Thyme Frittata* (page 218) **Lunch:** Orange Turkey Salad (page 220) **Dinner:** Celery & Cottage Cheese Beet Dip (page 221)	Calories:	1,565	Calories:	2,082
		Protein:	158g	Protein:	202g
		Carbs:	105g	Carbs:	134g
		Fat:	57g	Fat:	82g
SUNDAY	**Breakfast:** Golden Milk Chia Breakfast* (page 222) **Lunch:** Smoky Chicken & Corn Chowder (page 224) **Dinner:** Strawberry Protein Ice Cream (page 225)	Calories:	1,505	Calories:	1,984
		Protein:	145g	Protein:	183g
		Carbs:	94g	Carbs:	133g
		Fat:	61g	Fat:	80g

If you are following the 2,000-Calorie Plan, you will eat a double portion of this meal.

Instructions for slow-cooking the beef for the week ahead: Place 1 pound 7 ounces boneless lean beef in a slow cooker with 2 teaspoons salt, 2 teaspoons ground black pepper, 1 tablespoon dried rosemary leaves, and 1 clove garlic. Cook on low for 4 hours. Remove the meat from the slow cooker and shred with two forks.

Instructions for slow-cooking the chicken for the week ahead: Place 1 pound 7 ounces boneless, skinless chicken breasts in a slow cooker with 1½ teaspoons salt, 1½ teaspoons ground black pepper, 1 clove garlic, and 1 bay leaf. Cook on low for 4 hours. Remove the meat from the slow cooker.

Instructions for slow-cooking the turkey for the week ahead: Place 1 pound 7 ounces boneless, skinless turkey breast in a slow cooker with 2 teaspoons salt, 2 teaspoons ground black pepper, 1 clove garlic, and 1 bay leaf. Cook on low for 4 hours. Remove the meat from the slow cooker and cut into strips.

WEEK 2 SHOPPING LIST

*Additional quantities for the 2,000-Calorie Plan are marked with an asterisk.

MEAT, EGGS & DAIRY:

Boneless lean beef, 1½ pounds

Boneless, skinless chicken breasts, 1½ pounds

Boneless, skinless turkey breast, 1½ pounds, or 18 ounces turkey ham

Cottage cheese, low-fat, 3¾ cups (30 ounces)

Egg whites, 18 large, or 2¼ cups liquid egg whites (*add 18 large egg whites or 2¼ cups liquid egg whites)

Eggs, 6 large (*add 6)

Greek yogurt, plain low-fat, 6 cups (48 ounces)

FRESH PRODUCE:

Arugula, 12 cups (8½ ounces)

Bananas, 3 medium (*add 3)

Celery, 13 medium stalks (about 1½ bunches)

Corn, 1 ear

Garlic, 3 cloves

Granny Smith apples, 3

Kale, 3 bunches

Mushrooms, white, 1¼ pounds (*add 1¼ pounds)

Navel oranges, 3 (about 4 ounces each)

Orange juice, 3 ounces

Potato, 1 large

Red bell peppers, 3 medium (*add 3)

Thyme, 1 bunch

Yellow or white onions, 4 medium (*add 3)

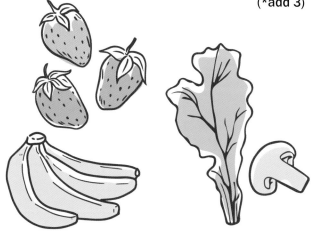

PANTRY & FREEZER ITEMS:

Almond butter, 5½ tablespoons (*add 1½ tablespoons)

Almond milk, unsweetened, 22 ounces (*add 6 ounces)

Apple cider vinegar, 1½ ounces

Beets, cooked, 15 ounces

Chia seeds, ¼ cup (*add ¼ cup)

Chicken stock, 1 cup

Cocoa powder, 3 ounces (*add 3 ounces)

Coconut milk, unsweetened full-fat, 3 ounces

Coffee, brewed, 24 ounces (*add 24 ounces)

Extra-virgin olive oil, 4½ ounces (*add 1½ ounces)

Honey, 2 teaspoons

Monkfruit sweetener, 1½ teaspoons

Nutritional yeast, 3 tablespoons

Prepared yellow mustard, 1¾ ounces

Strawberry halves, frozen, 1 cup (8 ounces)

Whey protein powder, 10¼ ounces (*add 7¼ ounces)

SPICES & SEEDS:

Bay leaves

Black peppercorns

Dried rosemary leaves

Garlic powder

Ground cardamom

Ground cinnamon

Salt

Smoked paprika

Turmeric powder

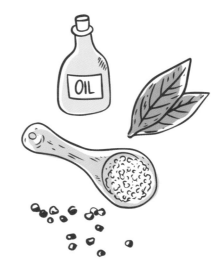

MON
TO
WED

MOCHA
PROTEIN SHAKE

FOR 1,500-CALORIE PLAN:

1 medium banana

1½ tablespoons almond butter

1 cup brewed coffee, chilled

2 ounces whey protein powder

2 tablespoons cocoa powder

FOR 2,000-CALORIE PLAN:

2 medium bananas

3 tablespoons almond butter

2 cups brewed coffee, chilled

4 ounces whey protein powder

¼ cup cocoa powder

Whiz all the ingredients in a blender. Pour into a glass and serve immediately.

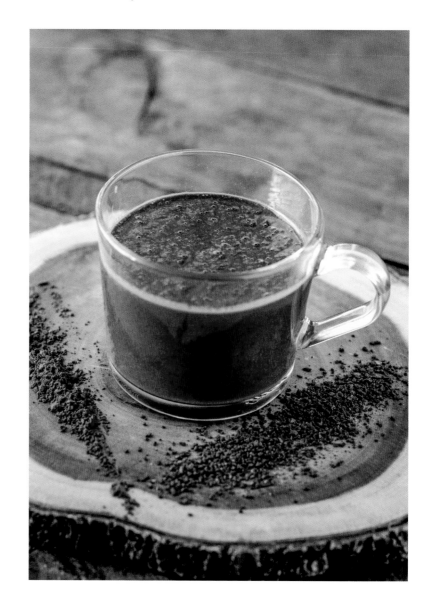

1,500-CALORIE PLAN:			
CALORIES:	PROTEIN:	CARBS:	FAT:
533	54g	41g	17g

2,000-CALORIE PLAN:			
CALORIES:	PROTEIN:	CARBS:	FAT:
1066	108g	82g	34g

ROSEMARY BEEF & "CHEESY" KALE SALAD

2 cups destemmed and chopped kale

1 tablespoon extra-virgin olive oil

1 tablespoon apple cider vinegar

½ teaspoon salt

½ teaspoon ground black pepper

1 tablespoon nutritional yeast

6 ounces shredded slow-cooked lean beef (page 211), warmed

Squeeze the kale a couple of times with your hand to soften it, then put it in a bowl. In a small jar, shake the oil, vinegar, salt, and pepper. Pour the dressing over the kale and mix well. Sprinkle with the nutritional yeast and serve with the beef.

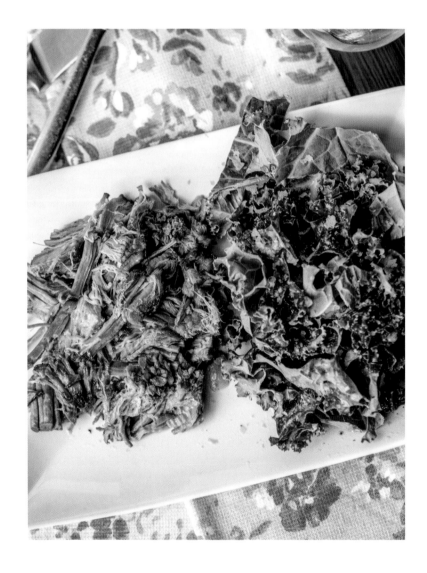

CALORIES:	PROTEIN:	CARBS:	FAT:
515	46g	15g	27g

MON
TO
WED

TART APPLE
CHICKEN SALAD

2 medium stalks celery

1 Granny Smith apple

5 ounces slow-cooked chicken breast (page 211), cut into bite-sized cubes

1 cup plain low-fat Greek yogurt

1 tablespoon prepared yellow mustard

½ teaspoon garlic powder

Salt and pepper

1. Cut the celery and apple into bite-sized cubes and place in a bowl. Add the chicken and toss to combine.

2. In another bowl, whisk together the yogurt, mustard, and garlic powder, then season with salt and pepper to taste. Add the chicken mixture to the dressing bowl and toss well.

CALORIES:	PROTEIN:	CARBS:	FAT:
532	67g	39g	12g

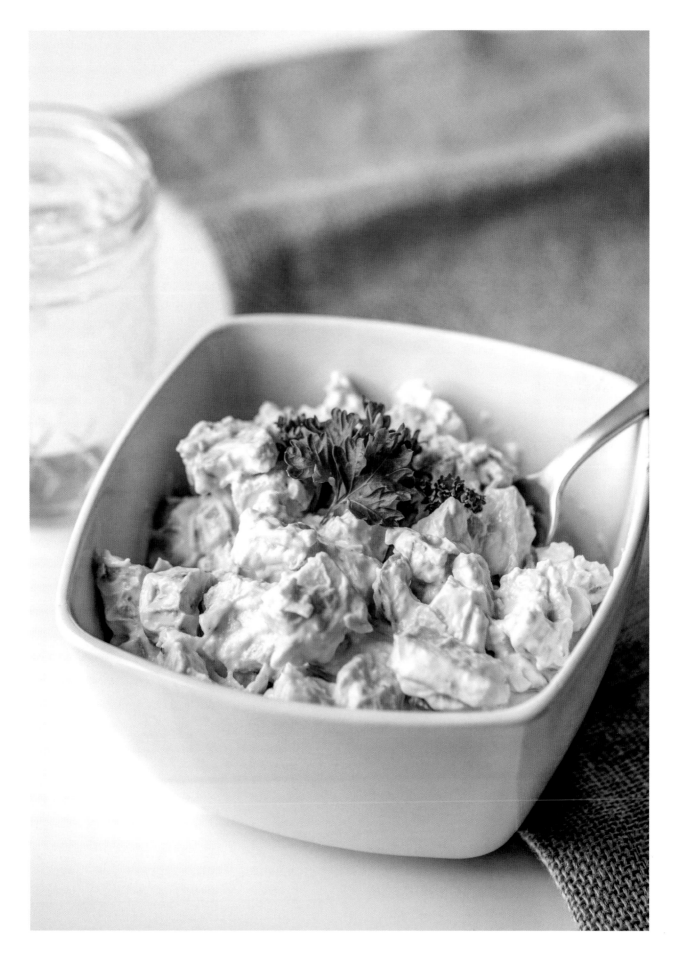

THU
TO
SAT

MUSHROOM, ONION
& THYME FRITTATA

FOR 1,500-CALORIE PLAN:

1 tablespoon extra-virgin
olive oil

1 medium yellow or white
onion, halved and sliced

1 medium red bell pepper,
halved lengthwise, deseeded,
and sliced

6 ounces white mushrooms,
sliced

1 tablespoon fresh thyme
leaves

Salt and pepper

2 large eggs

6 large egg whites, or ¾ cup
liquid egg whites

FOR 2,000-CALORIE PLAN:

2 tablespoons extra-virgin
olive oil

2 medium yellow or white
onions, halved and sliced

2 medium red bell peppers,
halved lengthwise, deseeded,
and sliced

12 ounces white mushrooms,
sliced

2 tablespoons fresh thyme
leaves

Salt and pepper

4 large eggs

12 large egg whites, or
1½ cups liquid egg whites

1. Heat the oil in a medium or large skillet (depending on which plan you are following) over medium-high heat. Add the onion(s), bell pepper(s), mushrooms, and thyme; cook, stirring frequently, until softened, 10 to 15 minutes. Season with salt and pepper to taste.

2. In a medium bowl, whisk the eggs and egg whites until homogeneous. Pour the eggs into the skillet and distribute the onion(s), pepper(s), and mushrooms evenly.

3. Cover with a lid, reduce the heat to low, and cook until the eggs are set, about 10 minutes.

1,500-CALORIE PLAN:

CALORIES:	PROTEIN:	CARBS:	FAT:
517	44g	21g	25g

2,000-CALORIE PLAN:

CALORIES:	PROTEIN:	CARBS:	FAT:
1034	88g	42g	50g

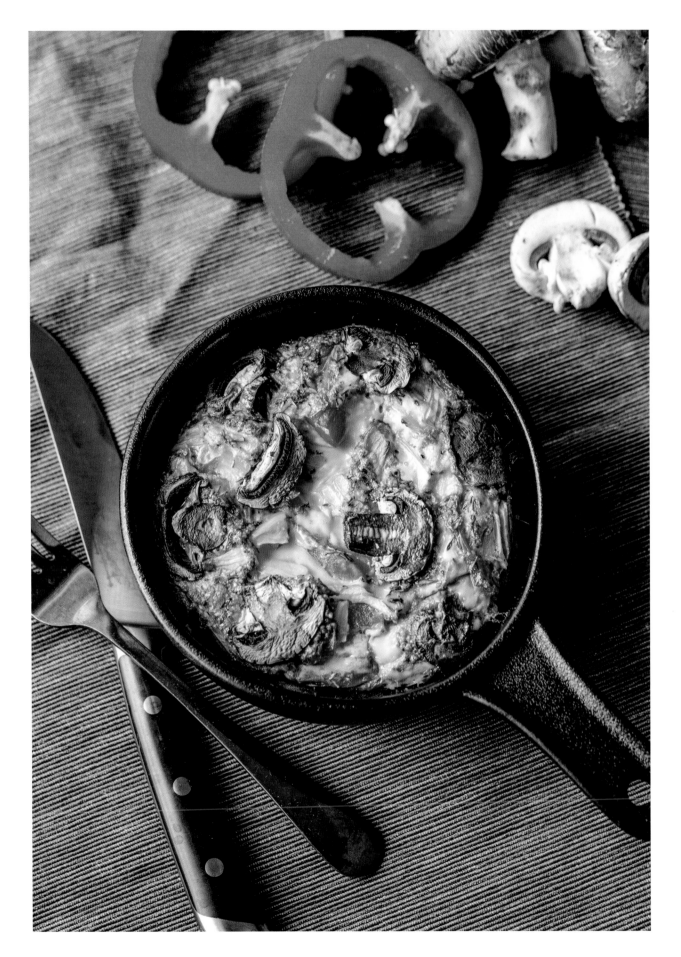

THU
TO
SAT

ORANGE TURKEY SALAD

4 cups arugula

1 (4-ounce) navel orange, peeled and cut into bite-sized pieces

6 ounces slow-cooked turkey breast (page 211) or turkey ham, cut into strips

DRESSING:

(Makes enough for 3 salads)

¼ cup plus 2 tablespoons orange juice

3 tablespoons extra-virgin olive oil

1½ teaspoons prepared yellow mustard

¾ teaspoon salt

¾ teaspoon ground black pepper

1. In a serving bowl, mix together the arugula and orange pieces. Arrange the turkey strips on top.

2. Put the orange juice, olive oil, mustard, salt, and pepper in a small jar and shake well to combine.

3. Drizzle one-third of the dressing over the salad and serve. (Store the leftover dressing in the refrigerator for use over the next two days.)

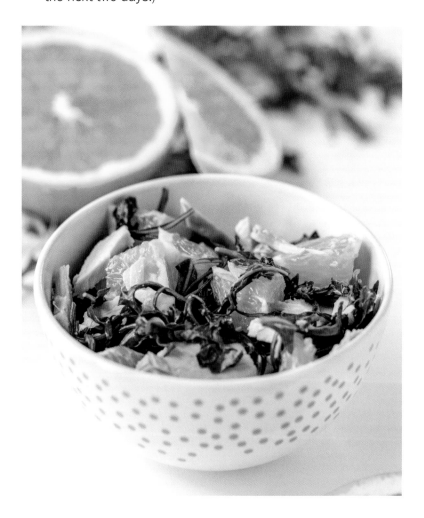

CALORIES:	PROTEIN:	CARBS:	FAT:
524	59g	36g	16g

CELERY & COTTAGE CHEESE BEET DIP

1¼ cups low-fat cottage cheese

1 cup plain low-fat Greek yogurt

5 ounces cooked beets

Salt and pepper

2 stalks celery, cut into 2-inch-long pieces

In a food processor, blend the cottage cheese, yogurt, and beets until fully combined and smooth. Season with salt and pepper to taste. Serve as a dip with the celery sticks.

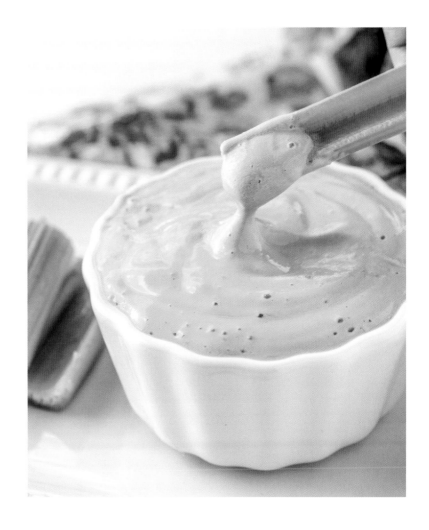

CALORIES:	PROTEIN:	CARBS:	FAT:
524	55g	40g	16g

SUN

GOLDEN MILK
CHIA BREAKFAST

FOR 1,500-CALORIE PLAN:

1¼ ounces whey protein powder

¼ cup chia seeds

½ teaspoon turmeric powder

¼ teaspoon ground cardamom

¼ teaspoon ground cinnamon

⅛ teaspoon ground black pepper

¾ cup unsweetened almond milk

2 teaspoons honey

FOR 2,000-CALORIE PLAN:

2½ ounces whey protein powder

½ cup chia seeds

1 teaspoon turmeric powder

½ teaspoon ground cardamom

½ teaspoon ground cinnamon

¼ teaspoon ground black pepper

1½ cups unsweetened almond milk

4 teaspoons honey

In a blender or food processor, blend all the ingredients until smooth. Add water if needed to achieve the desired consistency. Pour into a tall glass and serve immediately.

1,500-CALORIE PLAN:			
CALORIES:	PROTEIN:	CARBS:	FAT:
479	38g	39g	19g

2,000-CALORIE PLAN:			
CALORIES:	PROTEIN:	CARBS:	FAT:
958	76g	78g	38g

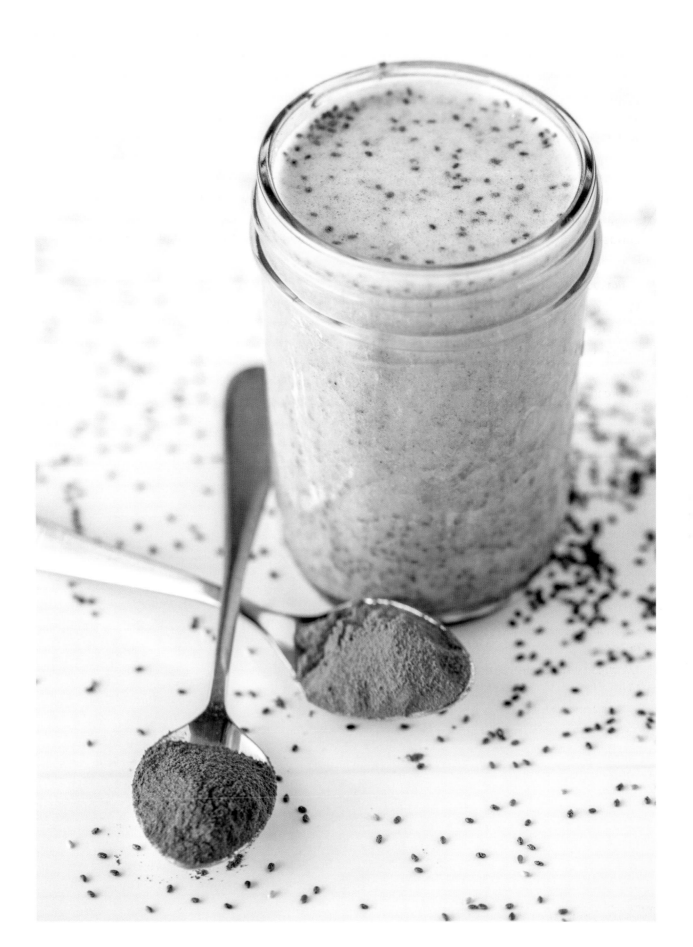

SMOKY CHICKEN & CORN CHOWDER

1 cup chicken stock

2 cups water

½ cup diced potatoes

½ cup fresh corn kernels

⅓ medium yellow or white onion, roughly chopped

¼ large celery stalk, chopped

1 bay leaf

½ teaspoon salt

½ teaspoon ground black pepper

3 ounces slow-cooked chicken breast (page 211), roughly chopped

⅓ cup canned unsweetened full-fat coconut milk

1 ounce whey protein powder

1 teaspoon smoked paprika

Put the chicken stock and water in a medium saucepan. Add the potatoes, corn, onion, celery, bay leaf, salt, and pepper. Cover with a lid and bring to a boil, then reduce the heat and simmer for 10 minutes. Remove from the heat, discard the bay leaf, and add the chicken, coconut milk, whey protein, and smoked paprika. Whiz everything with a stick blender until smooth. Adjust for salt and pepper and stir well before serving.

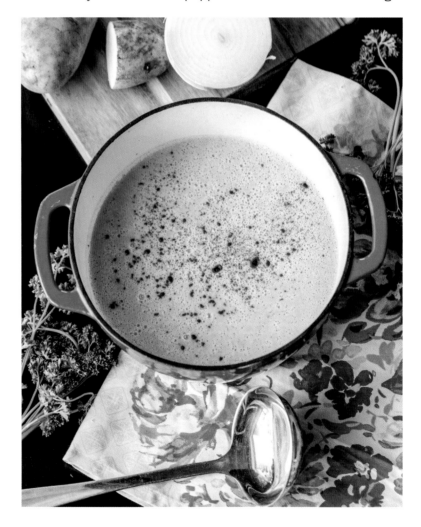

CALORIES:	PROTEIN:	CARBS:	FAT:
594	55g	30g	26g

STRAWBERRY
PROTEIN ICE CREAM

1 cup frozen strawberry halves

2 cups unsweetened almond milk

1 tablespoon almond butter

2 ounces whey protein powder

1½ teaspoons monkfruit sweetener

Put all the ingredients in a food processor and process until well combined. Transfer to a container and freeze for 30 to 50 minutes, until firm around the edges. Scrape and stir with a fork, then return to the freezer for another 30 to 50 minutes, until firm. Flake the ice cream with a fork again before serving.

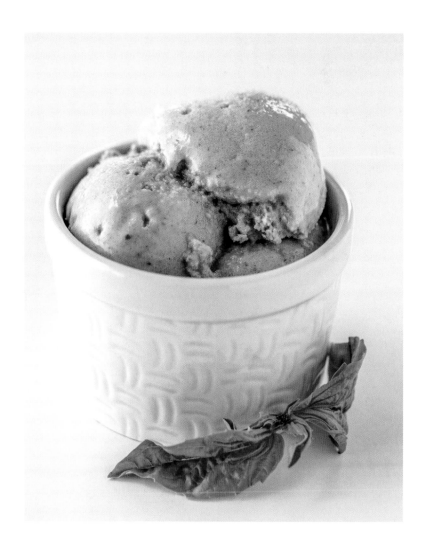

CALORIES:	PROTEIN:	CARBS:	FAT:
432	52g	13g	16g

		1,500-CALORIE PLAN		2,000-CALORIE PLAN	
MONDAY to WEDNESDAY	**Breakfast:** Omelet & Turnip Mash* (page 230) **Lunch:** Brown Rice Umami Salad (page 232) **Dinner:** Lemon Chicken with Sweet Potato Wedges (page 233)	Calories:	**1,522**	Calories:	**2,007**
		Protein:	**149g**	Protein:	**195g**
		Carbs:	**110g**	Carbs:	**138g**
		Fat:	**54g**	Fat:	**75g**
THURSDAY to SATURDAY	**Breakfast:** Mango Tuna Salad* (page 234) **Lunch:** Beef Steak on Parsnip Puree (page 236) **Dinner:** Pumpkin & Chicken Stir-Fry (page 238)	Calories:	**1,482**	Calories:	**1,909**
		Protein:	**167g**	Protein:	**212g**
		Carbs:	**109g**	Carbs:	**137g**
		Fat:	**42g**	Fat:	**57g**
SUNDAY	**Breakfast:** Cinnamon Protein Pancake* (page 240) **Lunch:** Veggie-Packed Lentil Soup (page 242) **Dinner:** Sweet Potato Puree with Crunchy Bacon Bits (page 244)	Calories:	**1,519**	Calories:	**2,018**
		Protein:	**138g**	Protein:	**191g**
		Carbs:	**145g**	Carbs:	**165g**
		Fat:	**43g**	Fat:	**66g**

If you are following the 2,000-Calorie Plan, you will eat a double portion of this meal.

Instructions for slow cooking the turkey for the week ahead:

Place 1 pound 9 ounces boneless, skinless turkey breast in a slow cooker with 1½ teaspoons salt, 1½ teaspoons ground black pepper, 2 cloves garlic, and 2 bay leaves. Cook on low for 4 hours. Remove the meat from the slow cooker.

WEEK 3 SHOPPING LIST

*Additional quantities for the 2,000-Calorie Plan are marked with an asterisk.

MEAT, EGGS & DAIRY:

Bacon, 3 slices

Boneless, skinless chicken breasts, 4 pounds 11 ounces

Boneless, skinless turkey breast, 1 pound 9 ounces

Egg whites, 30 large, or 3¾ cups liquid egg whites (*add 30 large egg whites or 3¾ cups liquid egg whites)

Eggs, 5 large (*add 5)

Ghee, 3 tablespoons (*add 3 tablespoons)

Grass-fed unsalted butter, 1 stick

Sirloin steak, 15 ounces

Sushi-grade tuna, 1½ pounds (*add 1½ pounds)

FRESH PRODUCE:

Arugula, 3 handfuls (*add 3 handfuls)

Banana, 1

Carrots, 6 large

Chives, 1 bunch

Cilantro, 1 bunch

Garlic, 2 cloves

Green bell peppers, 2

Leek, 1

Lemons, 2

Limes, 3 (*add 3)

Mangoes, 3 cups sliced (*add 3 cups)

Parsley, 1 bunch

Parsnips, 2 pounds

Potatoes, 2 large

Pumpkin or winter squash, 9 ounces

Red bell peppers, 2

Red onions, 2 medium

Sage, 1 bunch

Sweet potatoes, 2 pounds

Tomatoes, 2 large

Turnips, 2½ pounds (*add 2½ pounds)

Yellow or white onions, 2

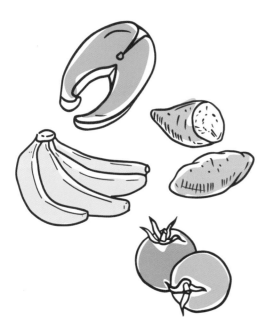

PANTRY ITEMS:

Baking powder, ½ teaspoon (*add ½ teaspoon)

Brown rice, 1 cup

Coconut aminos, 4½ ounces (*add 1½ ounces)

Cooking oil spray, preferably olive

Extra-virgin olive oil, 3¼ ounces

Green lentils, 13 ounces

Toasted sesame oil, 3 tablespoons

Whey protein powder, 6¾ ounces (*add 1¾ ounces)

SPICES & SEEDS:

Bay leaves

Black peppercorns

Coarse sea salt

Dried rosemary leaves

Dried thyme leaves

Fine sea salt

Ground cinnamon

Smoked paprika

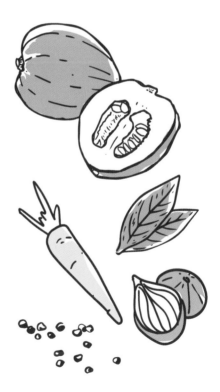

MON
TO
WED

BREAKFAST

OMELET &
TURNIP MASH

FOR 1,500-CALORIE PLAN:

13 ounces turnips, cubed

1 tablespoon ghee

½ teaspoon salt

½ teaspoon ground black pepper

1 large egg

10 large egg whites, or 1¼ cups liquid egg whites

Finely chopped fresh parsley, for garnish

FOR 2,000-CALORIE PLAN:

26 ounces turnips, cubed

2 tablespoons ghee

1 teaspoon salt, divided

1 teaspoon ground black pepper, divided

2 large eggs

20 large egg whites, or 2½ cups liquid egg whites

Finely chopped fresh parsley, for garnish

1. Put the turnips in a medium saucepan and cover with water. Boil over high heat until very soft. Drain, then puree the turnips with a stick blender until smooth.

2. Add the ghee and season with salt and pepper to taste. Blend again, adding a splash of water if needed to achieve the desired consistency.

3. Heat a large skillet over medium-high heat. Coat the skillet lightly with cooking oil spray. Whisk the egg(s) and egg whites in a large bowl until homogeneous. Stir in the salt and pepper and cook, covered, over medium heat until firm, about 10 minutes.

4. Serve the omelet with the turnip mash, garnished with parsley.

1,500-CALORIE PLAN:			
CALORIES:	PROTEIN:	CARBS:	FAT:
485	46g	28g	21g

2,000-CALORIE PLAN:			
CALORIES:	PROTEIN:	CARBS:	FAT:
970	92g	56g	42g

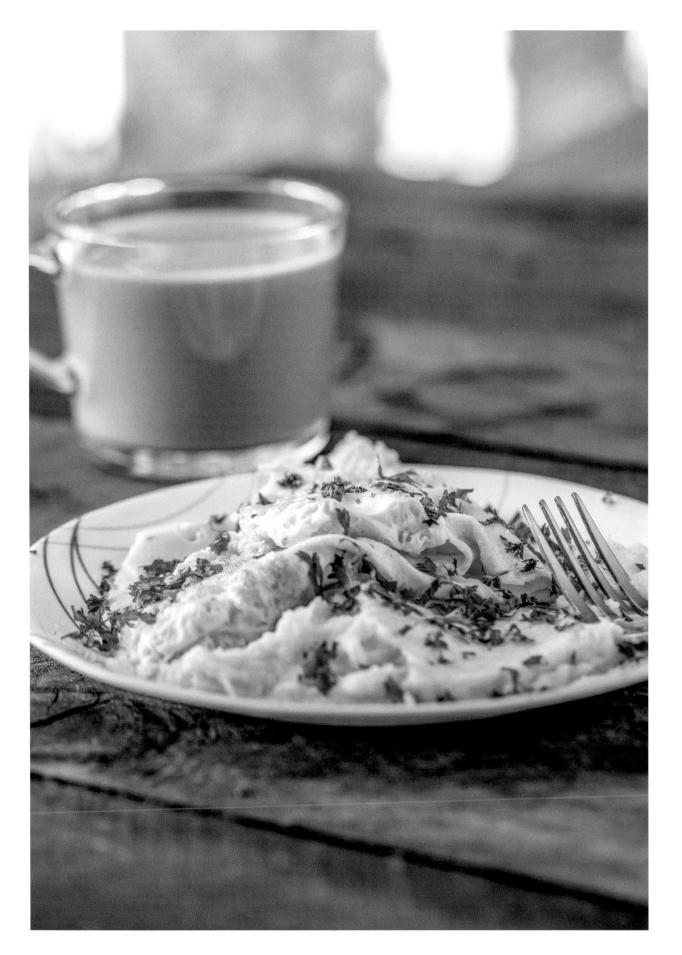

BROWN RICE
UMAMI SALAD

1 cup cooked brown rice, warmed

7 ounces slow-cooked turkey breast (page 227), diced and warmed

1 tablespoon toasted sesame oil

1 tablespoon coconut aminos

Salt (optional)

1 tablespoon chopped fresh chives

1 tablespoon chopped fresh cilantro

Combine the rice and turkey in a medium bowl. In a separate bowl, mix the sesame oil with the coconut aminos. Taste and add salt if needed. Drizzle the dressing over the rice and turkey and toss well. Top with the chives and cilantro. Enjoy warm.

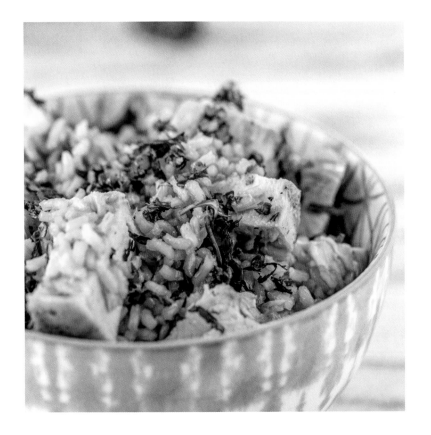

CALORIES:	PROTEIN:	CARBS:	FAT:
504	54g	36g	16g

LEMON CHICKEN
WITH SWEET
POTATO WEDGES

8 ounces sweet potatoes, scrubbed and cut lengthwise into wedges

1 tablespoon extra-virgin olive oil

1 teaspoon ground cinnamon

½ teaspoon salt, divided

½ teaspoon ground black pepper, divided

12 ounces boneless, skinless chicken breasts

1 tablespoon lemon juice

1. Preheat the oven to 425°F.

2. Put the sweet potatoes in a medium bowl. Add the oil, cinnamon, ¼ teaspoon of the salt, and ¼ teaspoon of the pepper; toss well.

3. Spread out the sweet potato wedges on a rimmed baking sheet and bake until golden brown, 30 to 40 minutes, flipping the wedges halfway through baking.

4. Meanwhile, grill the chicken over high heat until golden on both sides, about 15 minutes. Drizzle the lemon juice over the chicken and season with the remaining ¼ teaspoon each of salt and pepper. Serve with the sweet potato wedges.

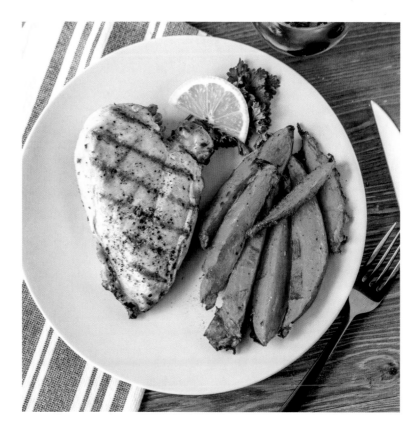

CALORIES:	PROTEIN:	CARBS:	FAT:
533	49g	46g	17g

THU
TO
SAT

MANGO
TUNA SALAD

FOR 1,500-CALORIE PLAN:

8 ounces sushi-grade tuna, cut into bite-sized pieces

1 tablespoon coconut aminos

Juice of 1 lime

1 handful arugula

1 cup diced mangoes

¼ teaspoon salt

¼ teaspoon ground black pepper

Finely chopped fresh parsley, for garnish

FOR 2,000-CALORIE PLAN:

16 ounces sushi-grade tuna, cut into bite-sized pieces

2 tablespoons coconut aminos

Juice of 2 limes

2 handfuls arugula

2 cups diced mangoes

½ teaspoon salt

½ teaspoon ground black pepper

Finely chopped fresh parsley, for garnish

1. Place the tuna in a medium bowl. Put the coconut aminos and lime juice in a small jar. Close the lid tightly and shake to combine. Pour the mixture over the tuna and allow to marinate for a few minutes.

2. Add the arugula and mangoes to the bowl with the marinated tuna and toss well to coat with the dressing. Season with the salt and pepper. Garnish with parsley.

1,500-CALORIE PLAN:

CALORIES:	PROTEIN:	CARBS:	FAT:
483	45g	42g	15g

2,000-CALORIE PLAN:

CALORIES:	PROTEIN:	CARBS:	FAT:
966	90g	84g	30g

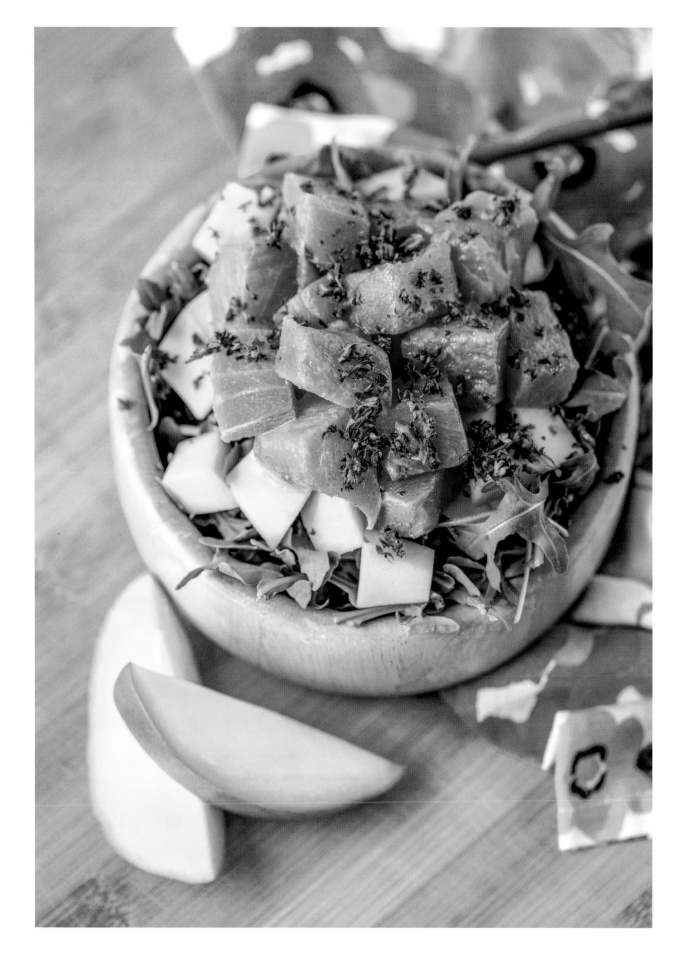

BEEF STEAK ON PARSNIP PUREE

10 ounces parsnips, sliced

1 teaspoon unsalted butter

1 ounce whey protein powder

¼ teaspoon salt

¼ teaspoon ground black pepper

4 ounces sirloin steak

Finely chopped fresh parsley, for garnish

1. Put the parsnips in a medium saucepan and cover with water. Boil over high heat until fork-tender; drain well, keeping the parsnips in the pan.

2. Add the butter and mash the parsnips using a stick blender. Stir in the whey protein and, if the puree is too thick, a splash of water. Season with the salt and pepper.

3. Preheat a gas grill to high heat.

4. Season the steak on both sides with salt and pepper and grill until browned on the outside but still pink inside, 2 to 3 minutes per side. Slice thinly against the grain and serve on a bed of parsnip puree. Garnish with parsley.

CALORIES:	PROTEIN:	CARBS:	FAT:
520	50g	53g	12g

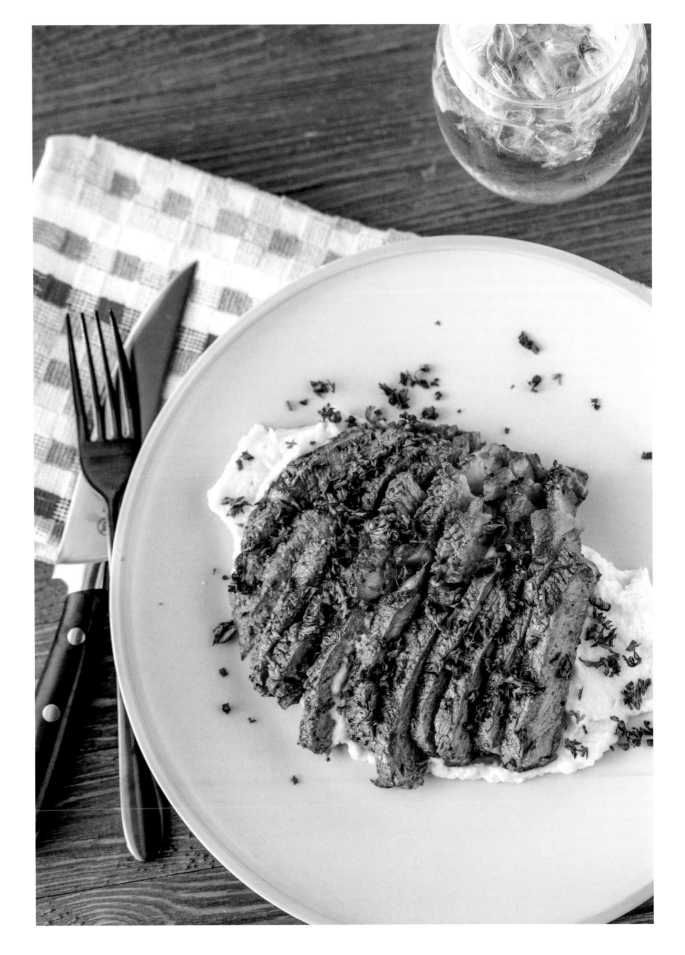

THU TO SAT

PUMPKIN &
CHICKEN STIR-FRY

1½ teaspoons extra-virgin olive oil

3 ounces peeled pumpkin or winter squash

½ medium red onion, cut into thick slices

8 ounces boneless, skinless chicken breasts, cut into thick strips

1 tablespoon coconut aminos

Fresh parsley sprigs, for garnish

1. Heat the oil in a medium skillet over medium-high heat, swirling the pan so the oil evenly coats the surface. Add the pumpkin and onion and stir-fry until golden, 5 to 7 minutes; then add the chicken. Cook, stirring frequently, until the chicken is cooked through, about 10 minutes longer.

2. Transfer the stir-fry to a serving bowl, dress with the coconut aminos, and garnish with parsley.

CALORIES:	PROTEIN:	CARBS:	FAT:
479	72g	14g	15g

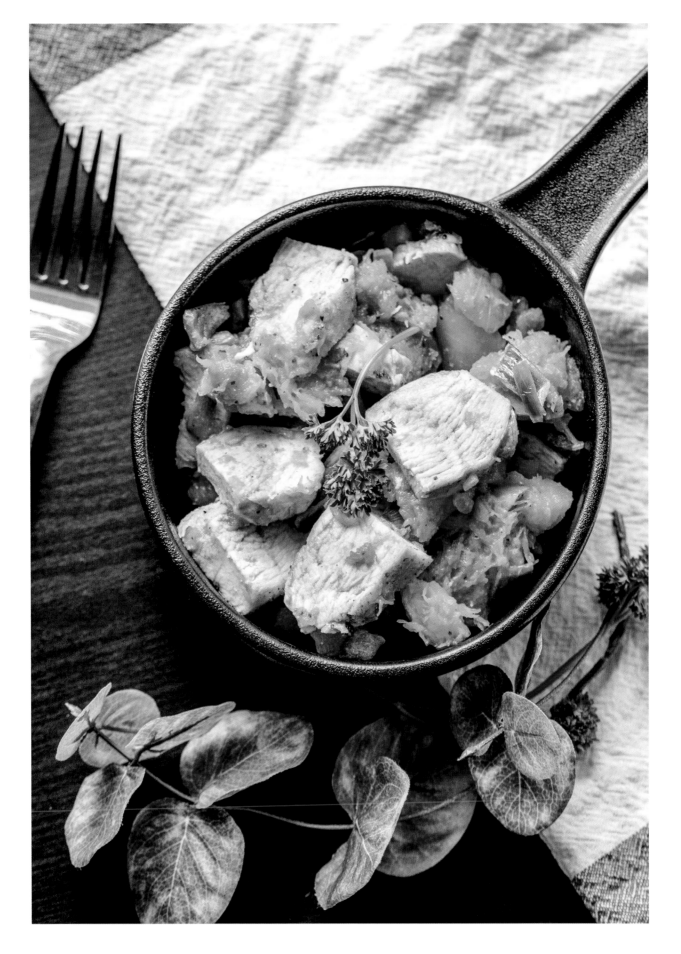

CINNAMON
PROTEIN PANCAKE

FOR 1,500-CALORIE PLAN:

2 large eggs

½ medium banana

1¾ ounces whey protein powder

1 teaspoon ground cinnamon

½ teaspoon baking powder

1 tablespoon unsalted butter, for the pan

FOR 2,000-CALORIE PLAN:

4 large eggs

1 medium banana

3½ ounces whey protein powder

2 teaspoons ground cinnamon

1 teaspoon baking powder

2 tablespoons unsalted butter, for the pan

FOR SERVING (OPTIONAL):

Banana slices

Sugar-free maple syrup

1. In a food processor, process all the ingredients except the butter until smooth.

2. Heat the butter in a medium skillet over high heat. Pour in the egg mixture, reduce the heat to medium, and cook until the pancake is firm enough to flip, about 2 minutes. Flip and cook until set on the other side, about another minute.

3. Transfer to a plate and serve warm. Top with banana slices and syrup, if desired.

1,500-CALORIE PLAN:

CALORIES:	PROTEIN:	CARBS:	FAT:
499	53g	20g	23g

2,000-CALORIE PLAN:

CALORIES:	PROTEIN:	CARBS:	FAT:
998	106g	40g	46g

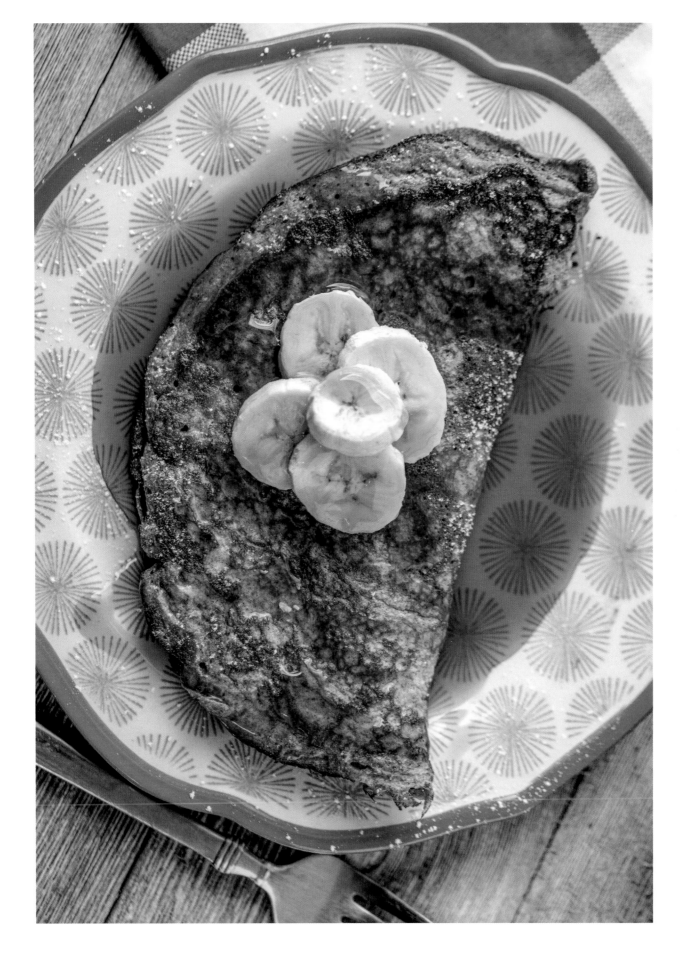

VEGGIE-PACKED
LENTIL SOUP

MAKES: *4 servings*

2 tablespoons extra-virgin olive oil

1 cup chopped yellow or white onions

2 cloves garlic, peeled

2 cups cubed potatoes

2 cups sliced carrots

6 ounces leeks, roughly chopped

1 cup diced red bell peppers

1 cup diced green bell peppers

2 large tomatoes, roughly chopped

1 teaspoon salt

1 teaspoon ground black pepper

13 ounces green lentils, soaked overnight or according to the package directions

1 large or 2 small bay leaves

1 tablespoon smoked paprika

1 teaspoon dried rosemary leaves

1 teaspoon dried thyme leaves

1. Heat the oil in a large saucepan over medium-high heat. Add the onions and garlic cloves and cook, stirring frequently, for 3 minutes. Add the potatoes, carrots, leeks, bell peppers, tomatoes, salt, and pepper; cook, stirring often, for 5 more minutes.

Add the lentils and bay leaves and cover everything with 2 inches of water. Bring to a boil, then reduce the heat and simmer, covered with a lid slightly ajar, for 1½ hours. Stir in the smoked paprika and taste for seasoning, adding more salt if needed. Remove and discard the bay leaves.

2. Stir in the rosemary and thyme. If you like, puree the soup with a stick blender until it reaches your desired consistency.

CALORIES:	PROTEIN:	CARBS:	FAT:
516	29g	82g	8g

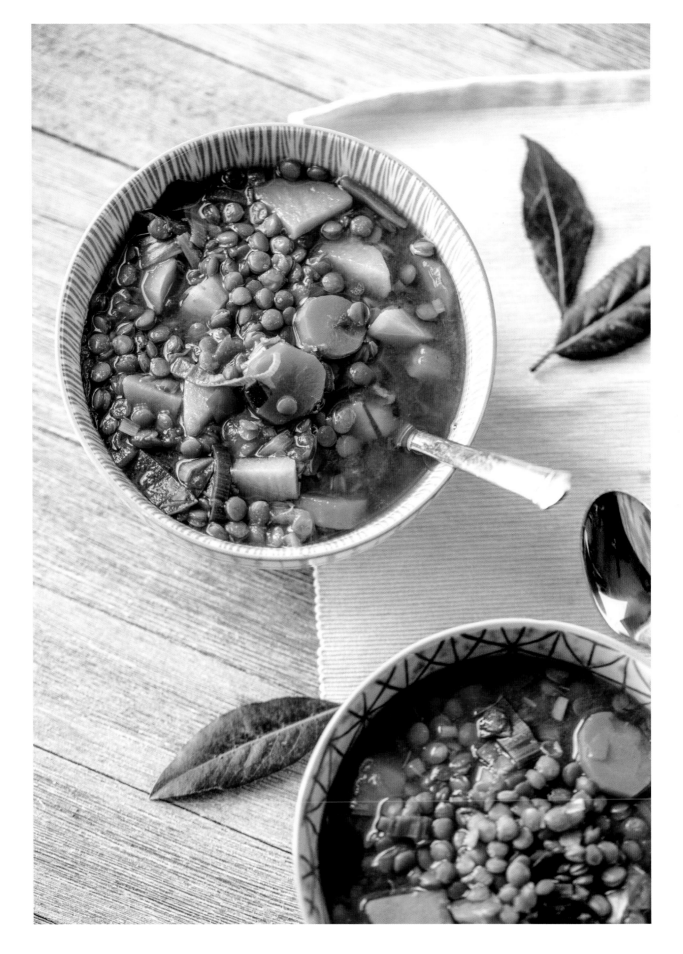

SWEET POTATO PUREE WITH CRUNCHY BACON BITS

SUN

7 ounces sweet potatoes, peeled and roughly chopped

3 slices bacon

2 ounces whey protein powder

½ teaspoon salt

½ teaspoon ground black pepper

1 sprig fresh sage, finely chopped

1. Put the sweet potatoes in a medium saucepan and cover with water. Boil over high heat until fork-tender, about 15 minutes.

2. While the sweet potatoes are cooking, fry the bacon in a medium skillet over medium-high heat until crispy, about 3 minutes.

3. Drain the sweet potatoes, keeping the potatoes in the pan. Add the whey protein, salt, and pepper and puree with a stick blender. If the mixture is too thick to blend, add a splash of water. Transfer the sweet potato puree to a bowl.

4. Crumble the bacon over the sweet potato puree. Sprinkle the sage on top and serve.

CALORIES:	PROTEIN:	CARBS:	FAT:
504	56g	43g	12g

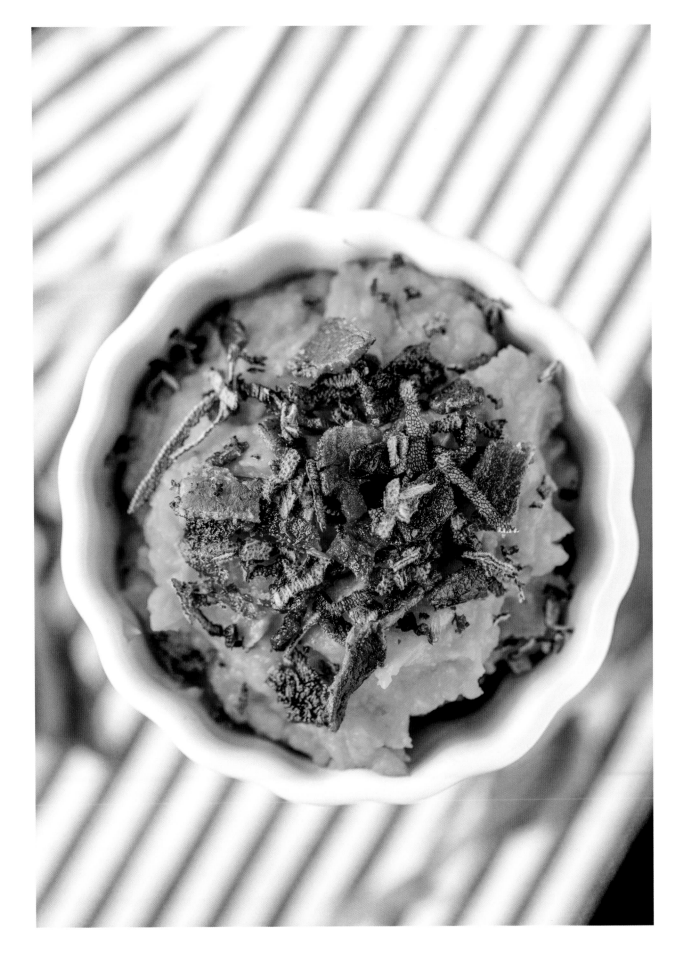

WEEK

4

		1,500-CALORIE PLAN		2,000-CALORIE PLAN	
MONDAY to WEDNESDAY	**Breakfast:** Mushroom Egg White Omelet & Sauerkraut* (page 250) **Lunch:** Spicy Tuna Poke Bowl (page 252) **Dinner:** Sweet Potato Boats with Smoky Shredded Chicken (page 254)	Calories:	**1,486**	Calories:	**1,977**
		Protein:	**152g**	Protein:	**222g**
		Carbs:	**125g**	Carbs:	**144g**
		Fat:	**42g**	Fat:	**57g**
THURSDAY to SATURDAY	**Breakfast:** Mango Green Protein Smoothie* (page 256) **Lunch:** Cinnamon Sweet Potato Fries with Lemon Yogurt Dip (page 258) **Dinner:** Cobb Salad (page 260)	Calories:	**1,514**	Calories:	**2,038**
		Protein:	**146g**	Protein:	**197g**
		Carbs:	**129g**	Carbs:	**200g**
		Fat:	**46g**	Fat:	**50g**
SUNDAY	**Breakfast:** Blueberry Protein Smoothie* (page 262) **Lunch:** Shrimp & Zucchini Bake (page 264) **Dinner:** Chicken & Lime Black Bean Soup (page 266)	Calories:	**1,454**	Calories:	**1,920**
		Protein:	**149g**	Protein:	**191g**
		Carbs:	**120g**	Carbs:	**172g**
		Fat:	**42g**	Fat:	**52g**

If you are following the 2,000-Calorie Plan, you will eat a double portion of this meal.

Instructions for slow-cooking the chicken for the week ahead:

Place 2 pounds 6 ounces boneless, skinless chicken breasts in a slow cooker with 1 teaspoon salt, 1 teaspoon ground black pepper, 1 clove garlic, and 1 bay leaf. Cook on low for 4 hours. Let cool, then remove and discard the bay leaf. Shred half of the chicken and cube the rest.

WEEK 4 SHOPPING LIST

*Additional quantities for the 2,000-Calorie Plan are marked with an asterisk.

MEAT, EGGS & DAIRY:

Boneless, skinless chicken breasts, 2 pounds 6 ounces

Egg, 1 large

Egg whites, 54 large, or 6¾ cups liquid egg whites (*add 30 egg whites or 3¾ cups liquid egg whites)

Grass-fed unsalted butter, 1 stick

Greek yogurt, plain full-fat, 5 ounces (*add 5 ounces)

Greek yogurt, plain nonfat, 17 ounces

Shrimp, large, 6 ounces fresh or 9 ounces frozen

Sushi-grade tuna, 18 ounces

Turkey bacon, 6 slices

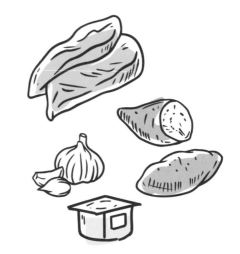

FRESH PRODUCE:

Bananas, 1½ medium (*add 1½ medium)

Cherry tomatoes, 12

Chives, 1 large bunch

Cilantro, 1 bunch

Cucumbers, 1 large or 2 medium

Garlic, 5 cloves (*add 3 cloves)

Jalapeño pepper, 1

Lemons, 2

Lettuce, 4½ cups (about 7 ounces)

Limes, 2

Mangoes, 3 medium (*add 3 medium)

Mushrooms, white, 1¾ pounds (*add 1¾ pounds)

Parsley, 1 large bunch

Red bell pepper, 1

Red onion, 1

Rosemary, 1 bunch

Scallions, 1 large bunch

Spinach, 6½ ounces (*add 6½ ounces)

Sweet potatoes, 9 medium (about 8 ounces each)

Thyme, 2 sprigs

Tomatoes, 3 medium

Yellow or white onion, 1

Zucchini, 1

PANTRY & FREEZER ITEMS:

Almond milk, unsweetened, 8 ounces (*add 8 ounces)

Arrowroot powder, 1½ teaspoons

Black beans, 1 (15-ounce) can

Blueberries, frozen, 11 ounces (*add 11 ounces)

Cooking oil spray (preferably olive)

Extra-virgin olive oil, 6½ ounces (*add 1½ ounces)

Monkfruit sweetener, 2 teaspoons (*add 2 teaspoons)

Nutritional yeast, 1 tablespoon

Primal Kitchen ranch dressing, 3 tablespoons

Salsa verde, 3 cups

Sauerkraut, 15 ounces (*add 15 ounces)

Sriracha sauce, 1 tablespoon

Tamari, 3 tablespoons

Toasted sesame oil, ½ teaspoon

Vanilla extract, 1 tablespoon (*add 1 tablespoon)

Whey protein powder, 10¼ ounces (*add 10¼ ounces)

White rice, ½ cup (4 ounces)

SEEDS & SPICES:

Black peppercorns

Black sesame seeds

Celtic salt

Chili powder

Crushed red pepper

Ground cinnamon

Ground coriander

Ground cumin

Smoked paprika

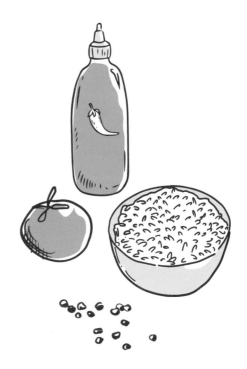

MUSHROOM EGG WHITE OMELET &
SAUERKRAUT

FOR 1,500-CALORIE PLAN:

1 tablespoon extra-virgin olive oil

9 ounces white mushrooms

10 large egg whites, or 1¼ cups liquid egg whites

1 ounce whey protein powder

2 tablespoons finely chopped fresh chives

2 tablespoons finely chopped fresh parsley, plus more for garnish

1 clove garlic

¼ teaspoon salt

¼ teaspoon ground black pepper

5 ounces sauerkraut, for serving

FOR 2,000-CALORIE PLAN:

2 tablespoons extra-virgin olive oil

18 ounces white mushrooms

20 large egg whites, or 2½ cups liquid egg whites

2 ounces whey protein powder

¼ cup finely chopped fresh chives

¼ cup finely chopped fresh parsley, plus more for garnish

2 cloves garlic

½ teaspoon salt

½ teaspoon ground black pepper

10 ounces sauerkraut, for serving

1. Preheat a large skillet over medium heat. When hot, add the oil and mushrooms; cook, stirring frequently, until the mushrooms are softened, about 7 minutes.

2. Put the egg whites, whey protein, chives, parsley, and garlic in a food processor and season with the salt and pepper. Blend until smooth.

3. Pour the egg white mixture over the mushrooms in the skillet and spread evenly. Reduce the heat to medium-low, cover with a lid, and cook until firm, about 10 minutes. Serve with the sauerkraut on the side, garnished with parsley.

1,500-CALORIE PLAN:

CALORIES:	PROTEIN:	CARBS:	FAT:
491	70g	19g	15g

2,000-CALORIE PLAN:

CALORIES:	PROTEIN:	CARBS:	FAT:
982	140g	38g	30g

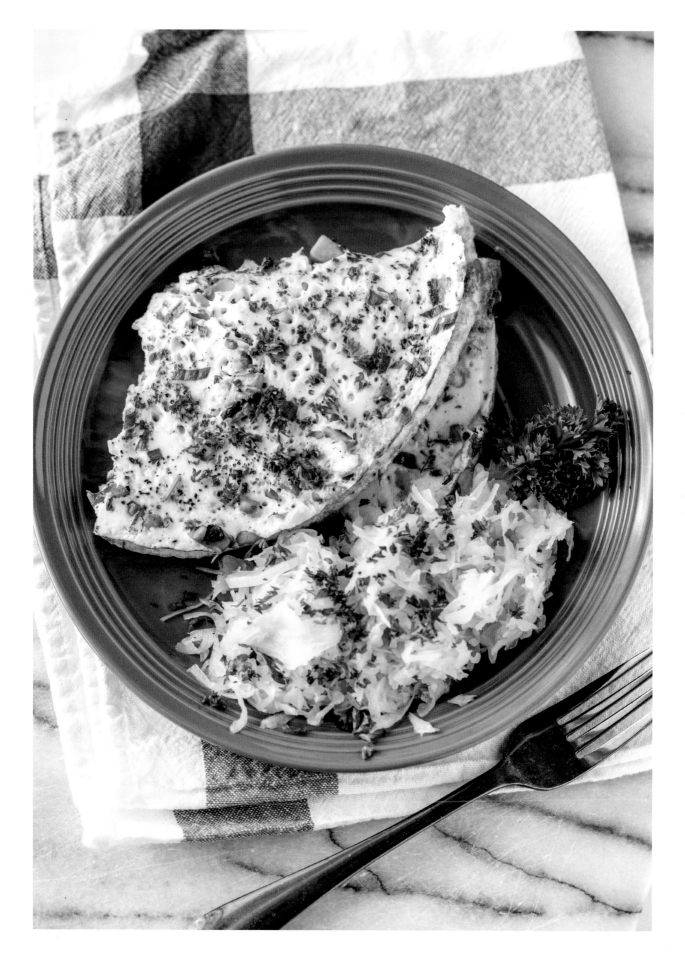

SPICY TUNA
POKE BOWL

1 tablespoon tamari

1 teaspoon Sriracha sauce

½ teaspoon toasted sesame oil

1 teaspoon black sesame seeds, plus more for garnish

6 ounces sushi-grade tuna, cubed

½ cup cooked white rice

½ cup sliced cucumbers

1 scallion, sliced

1. In a small bowl, mix together the tamari, Sriracha, sesame oil, sesame seeds, and tuna. Set aside to marinate for 10 minutes.

2. Put the rice in a small serving bowl. Gently stir the marinated tuna and place it on top of the rice; arrange the cucumber slices next to it. Sprinkle the scallion on top and garnish with sesame seeds.

CALORIES:	PROTEIN:	CARBS:	FAT:
484	45g	49g	12g

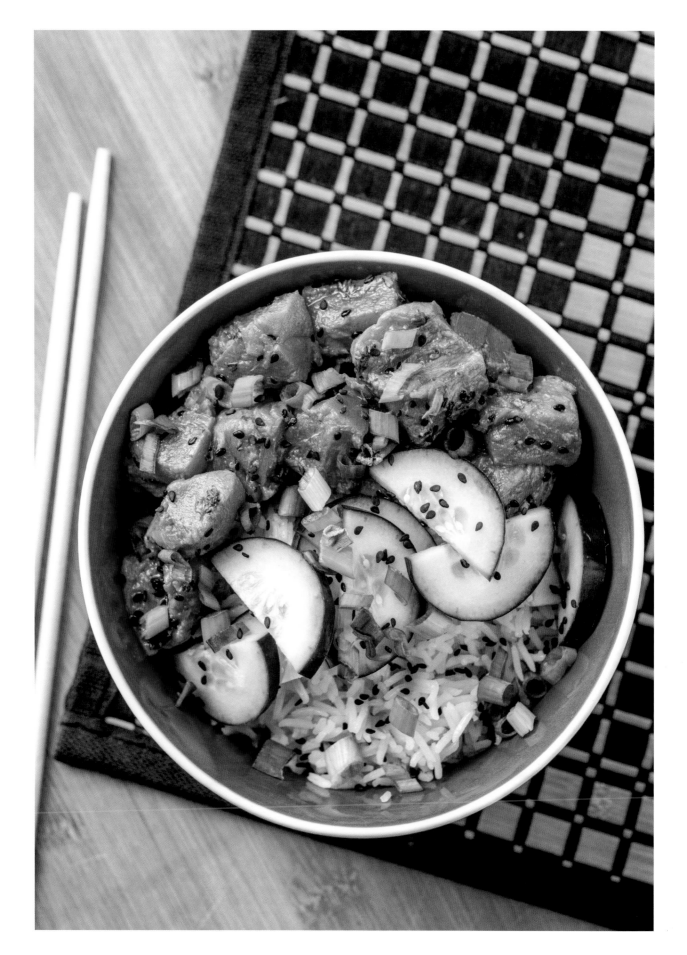

SWEET POTATO BOATS WITH SMOKY SHREDDED CHICKEN

MON
TO
WED

2 medium sweet potatoes (about 8 ounces each), scrubbed

4 ounces shredded slow-cooked chicken breast (page 247)

1 tablespoon smoked paprika

1 tablespoon extra-virgin olive oil

¼ teaspoon salt

¼ teaspoon ground black pepper

4 cherry tomatoes, halved

Finely chopped fresh cilantro leaves, for garnish

1. Preheat the oven to 400°F. Line a rimmed baking sheet with parchment paper.

2. Place the sweet potatoes on the prepared baking sheet. Bake until thoroughly soft, 30 to 40 minutes. Remove from the oven and let cool for about 5 minutes.

3. Once the sweet potatoes are cool enough to handle, slice halfway through them lengthwise and give them a gentle squeeze to open.

4. Warm the chicken and stir in the smoked paprika.

5. Drizzle the oil over the sweet potatoes, season with the salt and pepper, and then place the chicken on top. Top with the tomatoes and garnish with cilantro.

CALORIES:	PROTEIN:	CARBS:	FAT:
511	37g	57g	15g

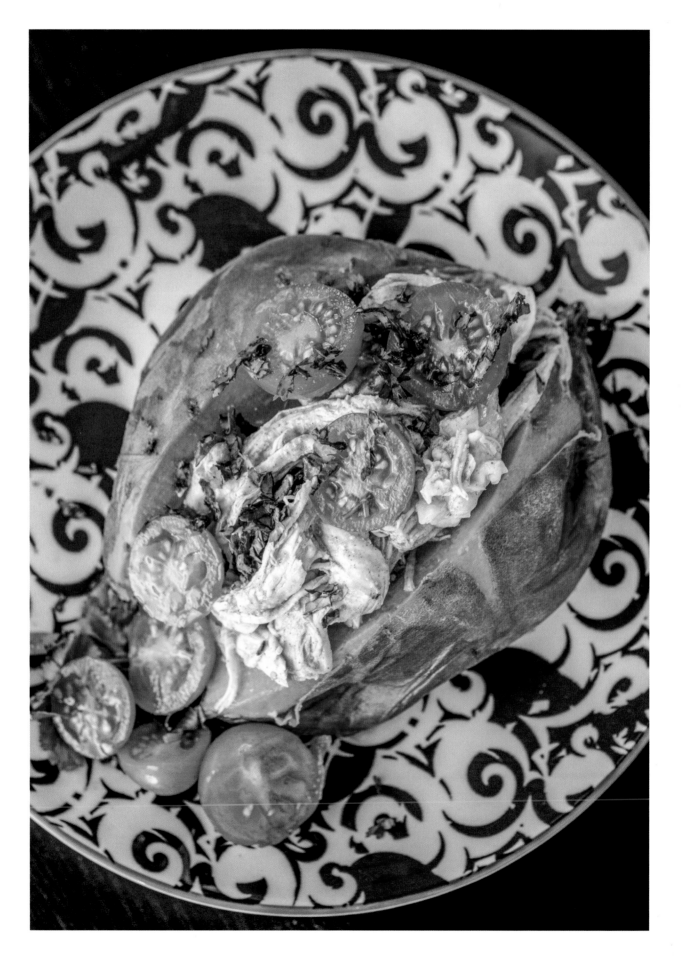

THU
TO
SAT

MANGO GREEN
PROTEIN SMOOTHIE

FOR 1,500-CALORIE PLAN:

2 cups fresh spinach

1 medium mango (about 12 ounces), peeled and cubed

½ medium banana

2 ounces whey protein powder

1 teaspoon vanilla extract

1 cup ice cubes

FOR 2,000-CALORIE PLAN:

4 cups fresh spinach

2 medium mangoes (about 1½ pounds), peeled and cubed

1 medium banana

4 ounces whey protein powder

2 teaspoons vanilla extract

2 cups ice cubes

Put all the ingredients except the ice in a blender and blend until smooth. Add the ice and whiz again. Add water if needed to achieve the desired consistency. Pour into a tall glass and serve immediately.

1,500-CALORIE PLAN:

CALORIES:	PROTEIN:	CARBS:	FAT:
524	51g	71g	4g

2,000-CALORIE PLAN:

CALORIES:	PROTEIN:	CARBS:	FAT:
1,048	102g	142g	8g

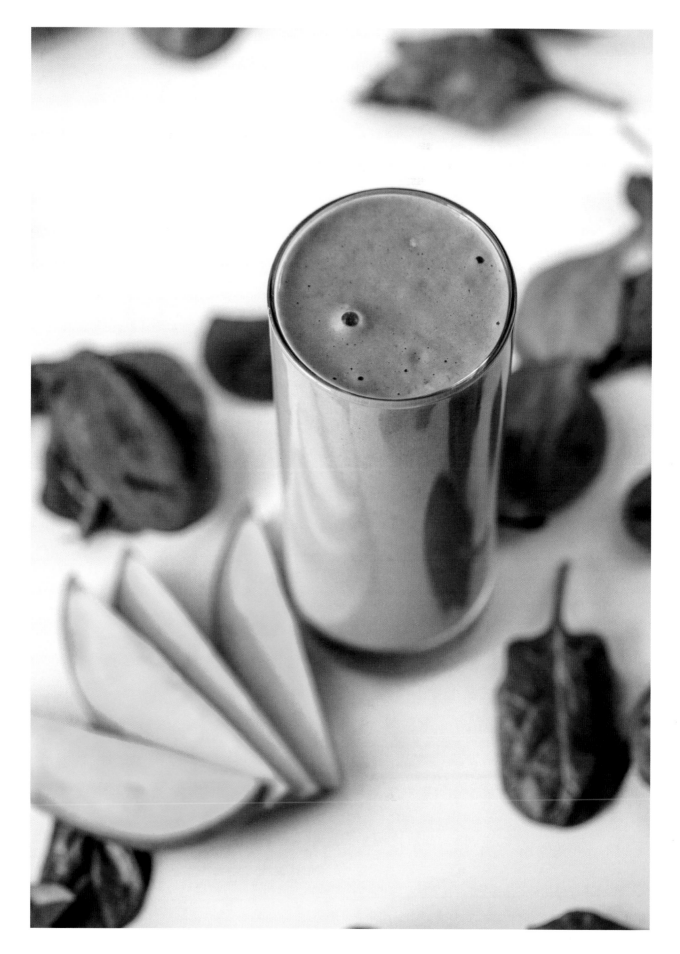

CINNAMON SWEET POTATO FRIES WITH LEMON YOGURT DIP

THU TO SAT

1 medium sweet potato (about 8 ounces), scrubbed

2 tablespoons extra-virgin olive oil

1 tablespoon finely chopped fresh rosemary

1 teaspoon ground cinnamon

¼ teaspoon salt

¼ teaspoon ground black pepper

LEMON YOGURT DIP:

½ cup plain nonfat Greek yogurt

1 tablespoon lemon juice

2 tablespoons chopped fresh chives

¼ teaspoon salt

¼ teaspoon ground black pepper

1. Preheat the oven to 425°F. Line a rimmed baking sheet with parchment paper.

2. Cut the sweet potato into wedges and place in a large bowl. Add the oil, rosemary, cinnamon, salt, and pepper and toss to combine.

3. Arrange the seasoned wedges in a single layer on the prepared baking sheet. Bake until golden brown, about 25 minutes, flipping the fries over halfway through.

4. Meanwhile, whisk the yogurt, lemon juice, chives, salt, and pepper in a small bowl. Place in the refrigerator to chill while the fries finish baking.

5. Serve the warm fries with the cool dip.

CALORIES:	PROTEIN:	CARBS:	FAT:
491	15g	47g	27g

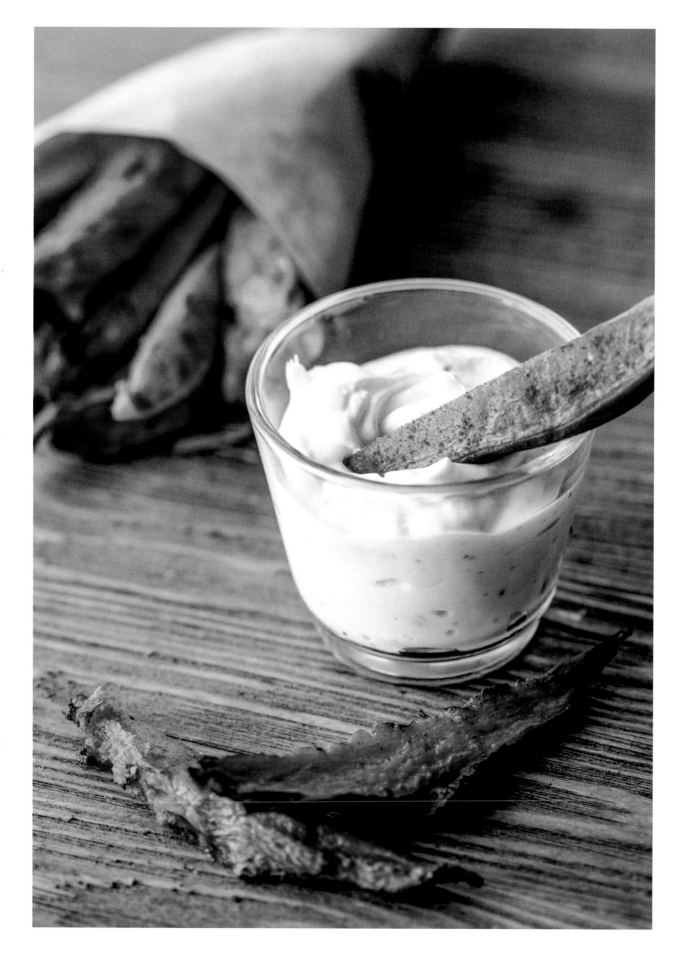

THU TO SAT

COBB
SALAD

8 large egg whites, or 1 cup liquid egg whites

¼ teaspoon salt

¼ teaspoon ground black pepper

2 slices turkey bacon, diced

1½ cups chopped romaine lettuce

5 ounces slow-cooked chicken breast (page 247), cubed

½ cup diced tomatoes

2 tablespoons finely chopped scallions

DRESSING:

(Makes enough for 3 salads)

¼ cup plus 2 tablespoons plain nonfat Greek yogurt

3 tablespoons Primal Kitchen ranch dressing

3 tablespoons water

1. In a medium bowl, whisk the egg whites until blended; then whisk in the salt and pepper.

2. Preheat a medium nonstick skillet over medium-high heat. When hot, add the turkey bacon and cook until crispy, about 2 minutes. Carefully transfer the bacon to a plate and set aside. Leave the bacon drippings in the skillet.

3. Pour the egg whites into the skillet, reduce the heat to medium, cover with a lid, and cook until opaque and firm, about 10 minutes. Remove the omelet from the skillet and let cool. Once cool, cut the omelet into ½-inch-wide strips.

4. Arrange the lettuce in a bowl or on a platter. Lay the egg white strips, chicken cubes, bacon, and tomatoes on top of the lettuce.

5. In a small bowl or jar, whisk together the yogurt, ranch dressing, and water. Drizzle one-third of the dressing over the salad and sprinkle with the scallions. (Store the leftover dressing in the refrigerator for use over the next two days.)

CALORIES:	PROTEIN:	CARBS:	FAT:
499	80g	11g	15g

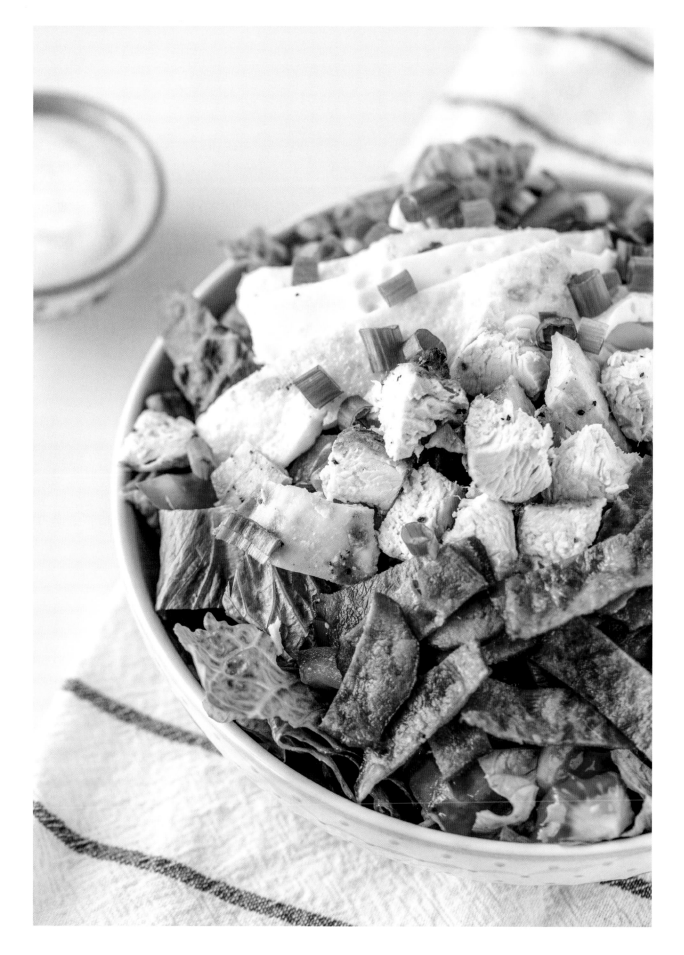

BLUEBERRY
PROTEIN SMOOTHIE

FOR 1,500-CALORIE PLAN:

½ cup plain full-fat Greek yogurt

2 cups frozen blueberries

1 cup unsweetened almond milk

2 teaspoons powdered monkfruit sweetener

1¼ ounces whey protein powder

FOR 2,000-CALORIE PLAN:

1 cup plain full-fat Greek yogurt

4 cups frozen blueberries

2 cups unsweetened almond milk

4 teaspoons powdered monkfruit sweetener

2½ ounces whey protein powder

Whiz all the ingredients in a blender, pour into a tall glass, and serve immediately.

1,500-CALORIE PLAN:			
CALORIES:	PROTEIN:	CARBS:	FAT:
466	42g	52g	10g

2,000-CALORIE PLAN:			
CALORIES:	PROTEIN:	CARBS:	FAT:
932	84g	104g	20g

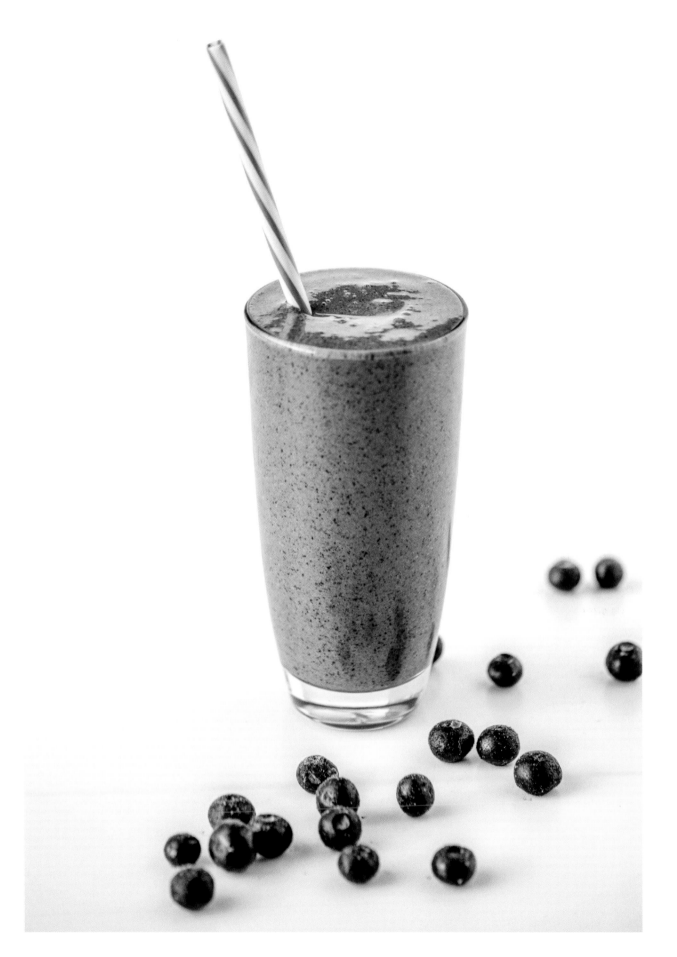

SUN

SHRIMP &
ZUCCHINI BAKE

¼ small red onion, diced

1 cup sliced zucchini

½ medium tomato, sliced

6 ounces fresh or thawed frozen shrimp, peeled

1 clove garlic, minced

1 large egg

1 tablespoon unsalted butter, melted, plus more for the casserole dish

1 tablespoon nutritional yeast

1½ teaspoons arrowroot powder

½ ounce whey protein powder

1 jalapeño pepper, thinly sliced

½ teaspoon salt

½ teaspoon ground black pepper

½ teaspoon crushed red pepper

Fresh cilantro leaves, for garnish

1. Preheat the oven to 350°F. Butter a small casserole dish or cast-iron skillet.

2. Sauté the onion in a small dry nonstick skillet over medium heat until fragrant, about 5 minutes. Layer the onion, zucchini, and tomato slices evenly in the bottom of the prepared casserole dish. Place the shrimp on top of the vegetables.

3. In a small bowl, whisk the garlic, egg, melted butter, nutritional yeast, arrowroot powder, and whey protein until the mixture is smooth. If it's too thick to pour, thin it with a bit of water. Pour the mixture evenly over the vegetables and shrimp in the casserole dish. Distribute the jalapeño slices on top. Sprinkle with the salt, black pepper, and crushed red pepper.

4. Bake until the veggies are tender and the shrimp are opaque, about 40 minutes. Transfer to a plate and garnish with cilantro.

CALORIES:	PROTEIN:	CARBS:	FAT:
499	64g	18g	19g

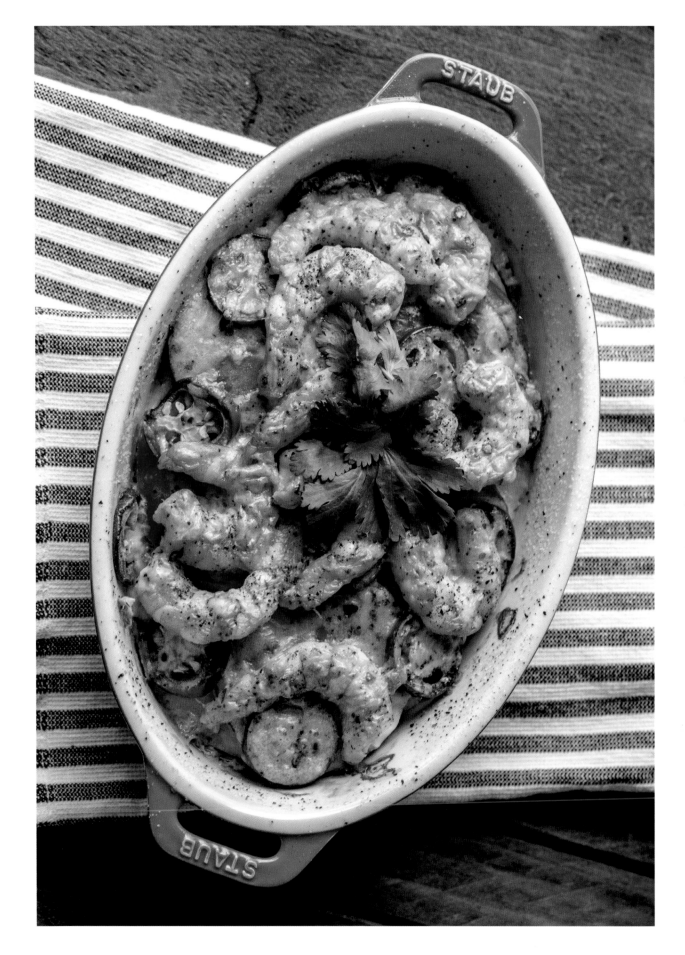

CHICKEN & LIME
BLACK BEAN SOUP

2 teaspoons extra-virgin olive oil

½ medium red bell pepper, deseeded and chopped

¼ medium yellow or white onion, chopped

⅔ cup diced tomatoes

1 clove garlic, minced

1 teaspoon chili powder, plus more for garnish

½ teaspoon ground coriander

½ teaspoon ground cumin

1 cup plus 2 tablespoons canned black beans, undrained

3 ounces shredded slow-cooked chicken breast (page 247)

1 tablespoon lime juice

1 tablespoon fresh cilantro leaves, for garnish

1. Heat the oil in a medium skillet over medium-high heat. When hot, add the bell pepper and onion and sauté until soft, about 10 minutes.

2. Add the tomatoes, garlic, chili powder, coriander, cumin, and beans with their liquid, plus ½ cup of water. Bring to a boil, cover with a lid, and simmer over medium-low heat for 15 minutes. If the soup becomes too thick, add a bit more water.

3. Put the shredded chicken in a serving bowl. Spoon the soup over the chicken, then stir in the lime juice. Garnish with the cilantro and a sprinkling of chili powder.

CALORIES:	PROTEIN:	CARBS:	FAT:
489	43g	50g	13g

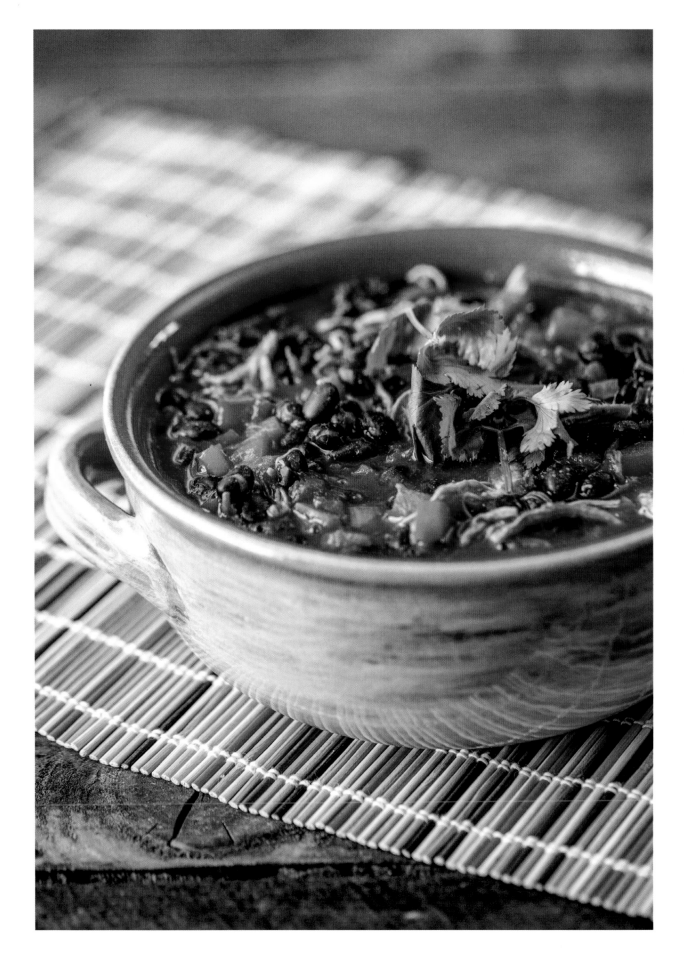

FOUR-WEEK BRING-BACK-THE-CARBS TRAINING PLAN

Monday	Lower Body + HIIT Cardio
Tuesday	Chest, Back, and Core + HIIT Cardio
Wednesday	Lower Body + Walking
Thursday	Shoulders, Biceps, and Triceps + HIIT Cardio
Friday	HIIT Circuit
Saturday	Upper/Lower Split + HIIT Cardio
Sunday	Rest

Please visit my YouTube channel for exercise demo videos: YouTube.com/coachtaragarrison.

UNDERSTANDING YOUR TRAINING PLAN

In each week of this plan, as your intake of carbs increases slightly, so will your reps and cardio intensity. Carbohydrates help support sustained intensity, so you will take advantage of the performance boost and train a little harder to make sure you put those carbs to work.

The weight you lift when doing these exercises should be heavy enough that it is difficult for you to finish the last rep while maintaining good form.

MONDAY: LOWER BODY + HIIT CARDIO

Warm up on the cardio machine of your choice for 5 minutes.

GOBLET SQUATS

Week 1	3 sets of 8
Week 2	3 sets of 10
Week 3	3 sets of 12
Week 4	3 sets of 15

ROMANIAN DEADLIFTS

Week 1	3 sets of 8
Week 2	3 sets of 10
Week 3	3 sets of 12
Week 4	3 sets of 15

STEP-UPS

Week 1	3 sets of 8
Week 2	3 sets of 10
Week 3	3 sets of 12
Week 4	3 sets of 15

LYING LEG CURLS

Week 1	3 sets of 8
Week 2	3 sets of 10
Week 3	3 sets of 12
Week 4	3 sets of 15

45-DEGREE HIP EXTENSIONS

Hold a plate to your chest to make this exercise harder if needed. Make sure to use your glutes, not your lower back.

Week 1	3 sets of 8
Week 2	3 sets of 10
Week 3	3 sets of 12
Week 4	3 sets of 15

SEATED CALF RAISES

Week 1	3 sets of 8
Week 2	3 sets of 10
Week 3	3 sets of 12
Week 4	3 sets of 15

CARDIO

Finish with 20 minutes of cardio intervals using the method of your choice. Warm up for 5 minutes, then repeat the following for 15 minutes:

Week 1	15-second all-out sprint followed by 2 minutes at a comfortable pace
Week 2	20-second all-out sprint followed by 2 minutes at a comfortable pace
Week 3	25-second all-out sprint followed by 2 minutes at a comfortable pace
Week 4	30-second all-out sprint followed by 2 minutes at a comfortable pace

TUESDAY: CHEST, BACK, AND CORE + HIIT CARDIO

Warm up on the cardio machine of your choice for 5 minutes.

DUMBBELL CHEST PRESSES

Week 1	3 sets of 8
Week 2	3 sets of 10
Week 3	3 sets of 12
Week 4	3 sets of 15

BENT-OVER SINGLE-ARM DUMBBELL ROWS

Week 1	3 sets of 16 (8/arm)
Week 2	3 sets of 20 (10/arm)
Week 3	3 sets of 24 (12/arm)
Week 4	3 sets of 30 (15/arm)

DUMBBELL CHEST FLIES

Week 1	3 sets of 8
Week 2	3 sets of 10
Week 3	3 sets of 12
Week 4	3 sets of 15

STRAIGHT-ARM LAT PULLDOWNS

Week 1	3 sets of 8
Week 2	3 sets of 10
Week 3	3 sets of 12
Week 4	3 sets of 15

SWISS BALL CRUNCHES (OR REGULAR CRUNCHES)

Week 1	3 sets of 8
Week 2	3 sets of 10
Week 3	3 sets of 12
Week 4	3 sets of 15

RUSSIAN TWISTS

A full twist to both sides equals one rep.

Week 1	3 sets of 20
Week 2	3 sets of 30
Week 3	3 sets of 40
Week 4	3 sets of 50

REVERSE CRUNCHES

Week 1	3 sets of 8
Week 2	3 sets of 10
Week 3	3 sets of 12
Week 4	3 sets of 15

CARDIO

Do 20 minutes of cardio intervals using the method of your choice. Warm up for 5 minutes, then repeat the following for 15 minutes:

Week 1	15-second all-out sprint followed by 2 minutes at a comfortable pace
Week 2	20-second all-out sprint followed by 2 minutes at a comfortable pace
Week 3	25-second all-out sprint followed by 2 minutes at a comfortable pace
Week 4	30-second all-out sprint followed by 2 minutes at a comfortable pace

WEDNESDAY: LOWER BODY + WALKING

Warm up on the cardio machine of your choice for 5 minutes.

LEG EXTENSIONS

Week 1	3 sets of 8
Week 2	3 sets of 10
Week 3	3 sets of 12
Week 4	3 sets of 15

SINGLE-LEG DEADLIFTS

Week 1	3 sets of 8/leg
Week 2	3 sets of 10/leg
Week 3	3 sets of 12/leg
Week 4	3 sets of 15/leg

SEATED LEG CURLS

Week 1	3 sets of 8
Week 2	3 sets of 10
Week 3	3 sets of 12
Week 4	3 sets of 15

BARBELL GLUTE BRIDGES

Week 1	3 sets of 8
Week 2	3 sets of 10
Week 3	3 sets of 12
Week 4	3 sets of 15

BARBELL GLUTE BRIDGES FROM FLOOR

Week 1	3 sets of 8
Week 2	3 sets of 10
Week 3	3 sets of 12
Week 4	3 sets of 15

STANDING CALF RAISES OR CALF RAISES ON LEG PRESS

Week 1	3 sets of 8
Week 2	3 sets of 10
Week 3	3 sets of 12
Week 4	3 sets of 15

GOBLET SQUATS WITH 3 PULSES

Week 1	3 sets of 8
Week 2	3 sets of 10
Week 3	3 sets of 12
Week 4	3 sets of 15

CARDIO

Walk as fast as you can for 30 minutes.

THURSDAY: SHOULDERS, BICEPS, AND TRICEPS + HIIT CARDIO

Warm up on the cardio machine of your choice for 5 minutes.

SEATED OVERHEAD DUMBBELL PRESSES

Week 1	3 sets of 8
Week 2	3 sets of 10
Week 3	3 sets of 12
Week 4	3 sets of 15

BICEPS CURLS

Week 1	3 sets of 8
Week 2	3 sets of 10
Week 3	3 sets of 12
Week 4	3 sets of 15

SKULL CRUSHERS

Week 1	3 sets of 8
Week 2	3 sets of 10
Week 3	3 sets of 12
Week 4	3 sets of 15

LATERAL L RAISES

Week 1	3 sets of 8
Week 2	3 sets of 10
Week 3	3 sets of 12
Week 4	3 sets of 15

BICEPS HAMMER CURLS

Week 1	3 sets of 8
Week 2	3 sets of 10
Week 3	3 sets of 12
Week 4	3 sets of 15

TRICEPS ROPE PUSHDOWNS

Week 1	3 sets of 8
Week 2	3 sets of 10
Week 3	3 sets of 12
Week 4	3 sets of 15

CARDIO

Do 20 minutes of cardio intervals using the method of your choice. Warm up for 5 minutes, then repeat the following for 15 minutes:

Week 1	15-second all-out sprint followed by 2 minutes at a comfortable pace
Week 2	20-second all-out sprint followed by 2 minutes at a comfortable pace
Week 3	25-second all-out sprint followed by 2 minutes at a comfortable pace
Week 4	30-second all-out sprint followed by 2 minutes at a comfortable pace

FRIDAY: HIIT CIRCUIT

For this circuit, you will perform each exercise for 30 seconds, rest for 30 seconds, and then move on to the next exercise. When you have completed all six exercises, rest for 2 minutes; then repeat the entire circuit two more times for a total of three rounds. Go hard or go home, baby! This entire workout is only 21 minutes long. When time goes down, intensity goes up. Get in, get it done, and get out.

1. Walking Push-Ups (or regular push-ups or push-ups with your hands elevated on a box)
2. Weighted Walking Lunges (heavy)
3. Battle Ropes
4. Squat Jumps
5. Wall Balls
6. Man Makers

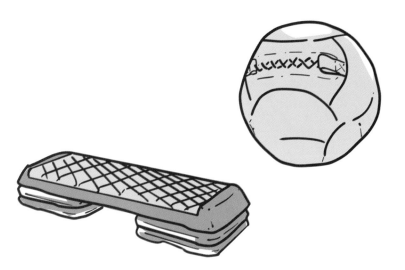

SATURDAY: UPPER/LOWER SPLIT + HIIT CARDIO

This workout uses supersets. That means you will do two exercises back-to-back with no rest in between exercises. Rest for 60 seconds between supersets. Follow the reps for the given week for all exercises.

SUPERSET 1

Lateral Raises with 5-Second Eccentric (take 5 seconds to lower slowly) and Reverse Lunges

Week 1	3 sets of 8
Week 2	3 sets of 10
Week 3	3 sets of 12
Week 4	3 sets of 15

SUPERSET 2

Alternating Biceps Curls and Romanian Deadlifts

Week 1	3 sets of 8/arm
Week 2	3 sets of 10/arm
Week 3	3 sets of 12/arm
Week 4	3 sets of 15/arm

SUPERSET 3

Triceps Kickbacks and 45-Degree Hip Extensions

Week 1	3 sets of 8/arm
Week 2	3 sets of 10/arm
Week 3	3 sets of 12/arm
Week 4	3 sets of 15/arm

CARDIO

Do 20 minutes of cardio intervals using the method of your choice. Warm up for 5 minutes, then repeat the following for 15 minutes:

Week 1	15-second all-out sprint followed by 2 minutes at a comfortable pace
Week 2	20-second all-out sprint followed by 2 minutes at a comfortable pace
Week 3	25-second all-out sprint followed by 2 minutes at a comfortable pace
Week 4	30-second all-out sprint followed by 2 minutes at a comfortable pace

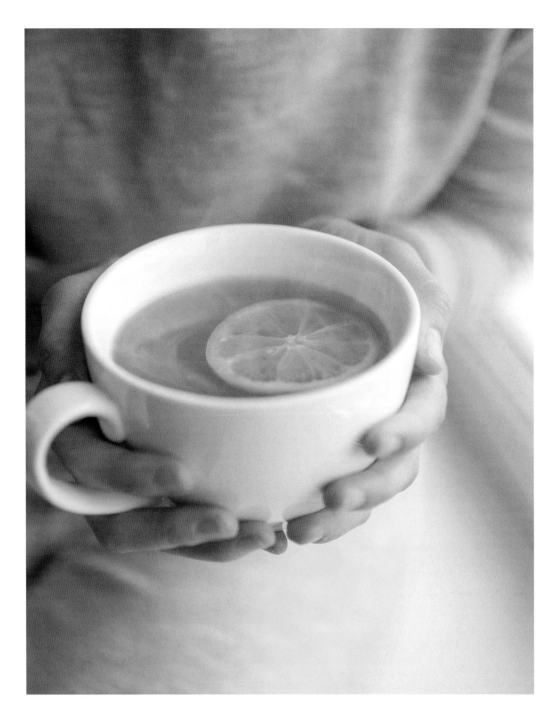

DISCOUNTS ON PRODUCTS

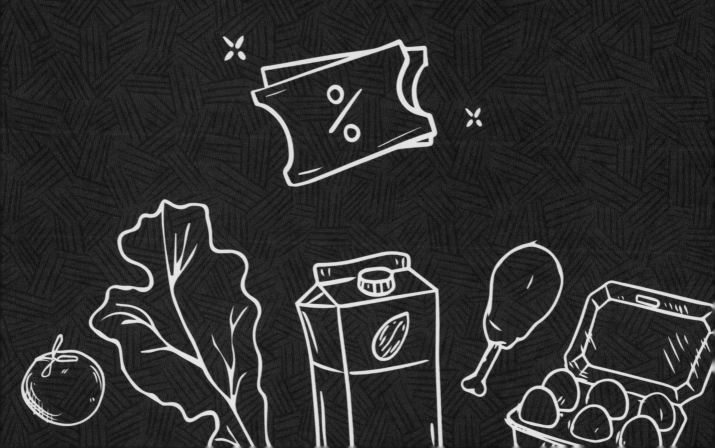

I only recommend products that I use and love, and I've asked the following companies for a discount for my clients and social media communities. As an affiliate for the following products, I receive a small percentage of sales when you use these coupon codes.

KETO MOJO BLOOD KETONE & GLUCOSE MONITOR

Website: ketomojo.com

Coupon code for 15% off: COACHTARA

UPGRADED FORMULAS HAIR MINERAL ANALYSIS & MINERAL SUPPLEMENTS:

Website: upgradedformulas.com

Coupon code for 15% off: INSIDEOUT15

HONEY BADGER SUPPLEMENTS (STEVIA-SWEETENED PRE-WORKOUT):

Website: drinkhoneybadger.com

Coupon code for 20% off: COACHTARA

ACKNOWLEDGMENTS

I would first like to thank my kids, Kenzie, Jarom, Kyle, and Micah, for supporting me in this wild ride of helping people and the planet.

I would like to thank Victory Belt for the opportunity to bring this book to the world and for all of the tremendous support during the creation process.

Thank you to Daria Gushchenkova and Ashtyn Blanchard for your help with the incredible recipes, to Karen Bethers for the recipe photos, and to Lyman Winn for the cover photo.

Thank you also to my many mentors/colleagues/friends, specifically Christian Thibaudeau, Shawn Wells, and Drew Manning, for your support and examples in my journey as a health professional.

And lastly, thank you of course to all of you who have purchased this book. It's my deepest desire to serve you in your health journey, because I believe health is the foundation of a happy and thriving life.

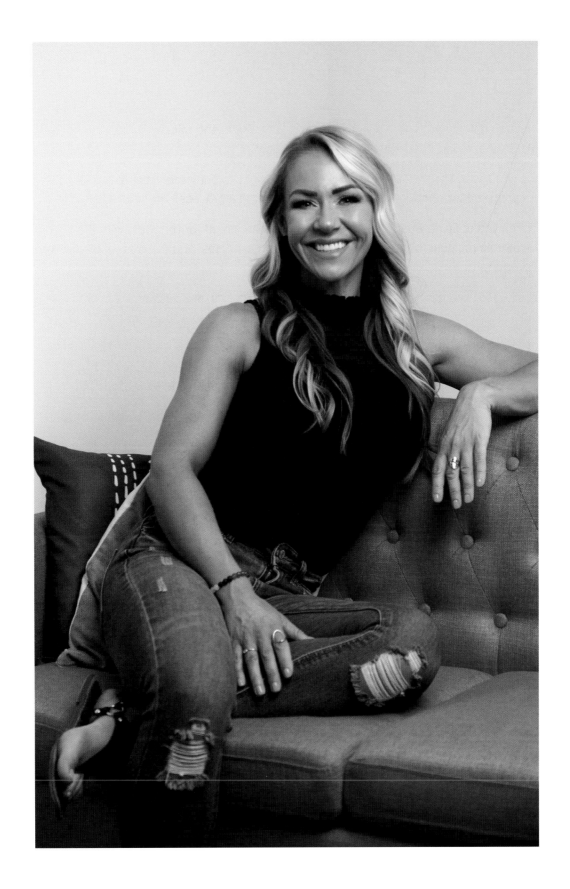

INDEX

Guacamole & Cheese Crackers recipe,
150–151

H

hair mineral analysis, 65
Halo Top brand, 50–52
HbA1c, insulin resistance and, 47–48
health conditions, keto and, 23–25
heavy cream
    Smoky Chicken Thighs & Creamed
      Spinach, 144–145
    Swedish Meatballs & Arugula, 168–169
High-Protein Niçoise Salad recipe, 200–201
Honey Badger Supplements, 277
Hong Kong, 84
hydration, 78
Hyman, Mark, 54–55

I

ice cream, 50–51
inflammation, keto and reduction of, 29
insoluble fiber, 68
insulin
    about, 105
    keto for reduction in, 30
insulin resistance, 45–55
intermittent fasting
    about, 107–108
    how to approach, 110–112
    research behind, 108–109
Italy, 91

J–K

jalapeño pepper
    Shrimp & Zucchini Bake, 264–265
Japan, 84, 85
kale
    Oregano Chicken with Wilted Greens,
      206–207
    Rosemary Beef & "Cheesy" Kale Salad,
      215
keto flu, 26
Keto Mojo Blood Ketone & Glucose Monitor,
    277
ketogenic diet
    about, 20–21, 54–55
    health conditions and, 23–25

length of time for, 38–41
long-term effects of, 42–44, 56–68
science-backed benefits of, 29–33
staying on, 93
therapeutic origins of, 22
ketosis, 23, 26

L

leeks
    Veggie-Packed Lentil Soup, 242–243
Lemon Chicken with Sweet Potato Wedges
    recipe, 233
lemons
    Baked Lemon Salmon & Asparagus,
      166–167
    Baked Turkey & Apples, 177
    Cinnamon Sweet Potato Fries with
      Lemon Yogurt Dip, 258–259
    Crispy-Skin Salmon with Cauliflower Rice,
      194–195
    High-Protein Niçoise Salad, 200–201
    Lemon Chicken with Sweet Potato
      Wedges, 233
    Zesty Chicken & Grapefruit Salad,
      148–149
lentils
    Veggie-Packed Lentil Soup, 242–243
lettuce. See romaine lettuce
limes
    Chicken & Lime Black Bean Soup,
      266–267
    Guacamole & Cheese Crackers, 150–151
    Mango Tuna Salad, 234–235
    Pulled Pork Tacos with Potatoes, 176
    Shredded Beef with Spicy Lime Quinoa,
      202–203
liquid egg whites. See eggs
liver, glycogen storage in, 42–43, 90
LowCarbUSA.com, 69

M

Mango Green Protein Smoothie recipe,
    256–257
Mango Tuna Salad recipe, 234–235
mangoes
    Mango Green Protein Smoothie, 256–257
    Mango Tuna Salad, 234–235

T